An Introduction to Practice Nursing:
The fulcrum of primary care

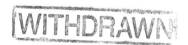

Also available in the *Issues for the Primary Care Team* series:

Travel Health for the Primary Care Team by Dr Mike Townend and Karen Howell
Eating Disorders for the Primary Care Team by Margaret Perry

An Introduction to Practice Nursing:
The fulcrum of primary care

Annette Bradley

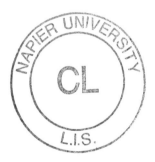

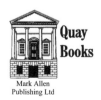

**Quay
Books**

Mark Allen
Publishing Ltd

Quay Books Division, Mark Allen Publishing Limited, Jesses Farm, Snow Hill, Dinton, Wiltshire, SP3 5HN

British Library Cataloguing-in-Publication Data
A catalogue record is available for this book

© Mark Allen Publishing Ltd 2002
ISBN 1 85642 214 3

Printed in the UK by Cromwell Press, Trowbridge, Wiltshire

Contents

Introduction

Ten years ago, on entering the unknown domain of practice nursing, one thing became apparent; the world of primary care and professional development was your oyster as long as you were prepared to learn to dive for it yourself. There was little written about the role, or how to succeed — after all, the role was very ill-defined at that time and differed from practice to practice and from area to area. Training was *ad hoc* and largely depended on the provision by the particular health authority to which the practice was responsible. General practitioners, practice staff and other health professionals were unsure of the knowledge and scope of practice nursing and could be forgiven for being unprepared for what lay ahead.

The role of the practice nurse is neither static nor well-defined; the role is changing from day-to-day as a result of changes locally, nationally and internationally. It can be argued that practice nursing is the fulcrum of primary care as we know it today, and probably tomorrow's leaders of innovation and development.

Practice nursing can be likened to a snowball, it keeps its original focus and aims but as it gathers momentum the snowball becomes bigger. If knowledge, support, training, education and professional development are inadequate to encompass this there is a danger that practice nurses will be overwhelmed by it and left behind.

This book will help nurses who are considering a move into general practice, nurses in an alternative setting or those involved with the commissioning or delivery of training to understand the culture and the role of practice nursing. It explains the meaning of the many words, jargon and definitions that are often heard in the primary care domain, which in a previous role have served a different meaning or have been of no relevance.

The first chapter gives an introduction to general practice and an insight into its culture and principles and those of practice nursing. It equips a nurse entering general practice with information and questions, from the interview process through to the induction period.

Training and education is an important part of being a competent and safe practitioner and *Chapter 2* explores the concepts of training, education and support in general practice nursing, including a model to be used by both mentor and mentee in the induction period. This chapter also includes an introduction to reflective practice and clinical supervision and the logistics and importance of these concepts in practice nursing, especially when practising in isolation from other practice nurses.

Further chapters include giving a whistle-stop tour of the latest political developments within the NHS, especially in relation to general practice and practice nursing and in providing practical skills in the area of setting up clinics, developing protocols and audit.

Finally, *Chapter 5* explores the future of practice nursing and how it may be marketed. It demonstrates the importance of innovation within the role and how practice nurses may develop as a result.

By providing a step-by-step detailed guide for nurses in all aspects of role and career development in general practice, the book will encourage those nurses considering a career in practice to become pro-active, competent practitioners rather than reactive pawns in a very competitive field.

Annette Bradley
February 2002

1

An introduction to general practice

Introduction

General practice is the linchpin of primary care, the gateway for the public to access primary care services. It has traditionally been the first port of call for the general public when sick and injured; however, with the development of triage services such as the NHS walk-in centres and NHS Direct, the characteristic gatekeeper function of general practice is changing. Many of the triage services are now being developed, managed and run by nurses: nurses are becoming the gatekeepers of primary care.

This chapter informs those nurses wishing to know more about general practice and general practice nursing, about its culture and role. It enables those nurses who want to enter general practice nursing to understand the application, interview and appointment procedure — while giving hints and tips on how to survive it.

Nurses working within general practice need to become confident, skilled practitioners as soon as possible in order to manage their own case-load competently.

What is general practice?

General practice usually consists of a health team of general practitioners, practice nurses and administrative staff who work alongside a supporting primary healthcare team (*Figure 1.1*).

Since the introduction of the personal medical services (PMS) pilots, as a result of the Government's White Paper, *The new NHS — modern, dependable* (Department of Health [DoH], 1997), the traditional picture of general practice is changing. These changes and opportunities for practice nurses are discussed in *Chapter 3*.

The list size of a general practice depends on the number of partners within it, usually around 2,000 patients per general practitioner or 10,000 per group of five (Fry, 1992); and in any one year it is estimated that 70% of those patients will consult their GP.

There are many single-handed general practitioners who employ only one practice nurse and who are not part of a health centre. Nurses working for such practices are often isolated from other similar professionals, which makes it important for them to be involved in the available support networks for practice nurses, eg. local groups, clinical supervision and mentorship.

Nurses employed within general practice are usually state registered or registered general nurses with a few being enrolled nurses, employed by general practitioners to complement the health-care team in the practice. Since 1977, the number of nurses has risen in general practice, most of them being female (Atkin and Lunt, 1993). With the introduction of the 1990 White Paper, *Working for Patients* (DoH, 1990), the numbers in general practice rose even higher as nurses were able to undertake much of the extra responsibility given to general practitioners as a result of the Government legislation. Indeed, Richardson *et al* (1995) suggested that 30–70% of tasks carried out by general practitioners could be carried out by nurses.

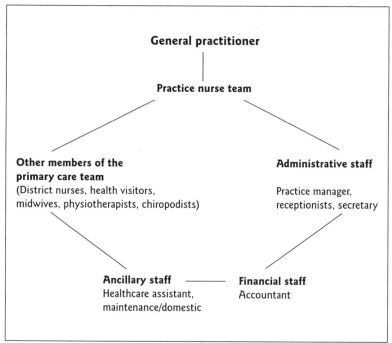

Figure 1.1: A typical traditional general practice team

Role of the practice nurse

She who controlleth the gate controlleth it all.

Diers and Molde, 1982

It is never going to be easy to define the role of the practice nurse, but one thing certain is that the role is challenging, demanding, evolving and exciting. For those who wish to further their career and prospects, practice nursing is an area to consider.

Traditionally, of course, it was a 'what does doctor want me to do for you' role, a supporting role for the general practitioner with little autonomy. Many women chose to go into general practice to suit family needs, with most positions being part-time and split shifts. This was reflected in a study carried out in Gateshead where the majority of practice nurses surveyed in 1980 were between the ages of thirty and forty-four and averaged working hours of twenty-two and a half per week (Reedy *et al*, 1980). The role was very often described as one of 'hand maiden' to the general practitioner (GP), and followed the medical model of care. With fewer nurses in general practice it would have been very rare for practice nurses to take a lead role within the practice. Within ten years and among many Government changes it has developed into a role that can arguably be one of the most important in primary care.

Government pressure to improve the cost effectiveness of primary healthcare provision has meant that care has been shifting from being provided by general practitioners to nurses (Richardson, 1995).

Other factors that may contribute to the shift are increasing retirement rates of GPs, declining recruitment and a shift towards the opportunities for part-time working in medicine.

To illustrate how much the role has evolved in the last thirty years it is worth comparing the tasks that Reedy (1972) found doctors delegating to nurses in a number of surgeries, ie. a limited list of blood pressure readings, escorting doctors, testing urine samples and weighing patients, to the tasks undertaken by practice nurses in the twenty-first century. Most of the tasks are now part of the accepted role of the practice nurse today. Tasks most commonly considered as the 'extended' role of the nurse in 1988 such as venepuncture, immunisations and vaccinations and cervical smears, are now usually encompassed in the practice nurse role. Bolden and Tackle (1984) wrote a handbook for practice nurses and in it highlighted that practice nurses could see asthma patients in the presence of a general practitioner. Now, of course, most practice nurses are asthma trained and often run clinics on their own.

The practice nurse role encompasses many dimensions (*Table 1.1*) and it is unlikely that a nurse entering practice from another domain of nursing would be adequately trained and competent to undertake all of the illustrated aspects of the role without comprehensive training and support.

Table 1.1: The dimensions of practice nursing	
Clinical	**Non-clinical**
Smoking cessation	Audit
Travel health	Team leader
Ear care	Use of information technology
Immunisations	Developing protocols
Health promotion	Developing practice profile
First aid	Clinical supervisor
Diabetes	Teacher
Coronary heart disease prevention	Researcher
ECG	Health needs assessment
Venepuncture	Representative of primary care group
Screening	Mentor/preceptor
Women's health	Report writing
Helping people change	Publishing works
Men's health	Record keeping
Wound care	
Asthma	

Research has shown that over three-quarters of nurses entering general practice are unable to carry out the role without a great deal of support and training from their colleagues (Bradley, 1998). Many nurses entering general practice have come from the acute setting and may find themselves in a role that is isolated with responsibilities for which they have not been prepared.

It is difficult to define nurse competence and whether a nurse is adequately prepared for the practice nurse role. Despite formal codes of competence laid down by the United Kingdom Central Council for Nursing, Midwifery and Health Visiting (UKCC; now known as the Nursing and Midwifery Council [NMC]), Bradshaw (1998) argued that when examining nurse competence in general they were not enough, and that there should be defined national minimum measurable standards for theoretical and practical competence for all nurses. The evidence from the research (Bradley, 1998) showed that competency of nurses entering practice nursing varies, suggesting that those minimum standards should also be used when nurses change their specialist area.

Table 1.2 illustrates typical examples of minimum, measurable competencies that may be adapted when a nurse enters general practice. It can be seen that the role not only involves clinical tasks, but also has a managerial and developmental side. It may be argued, that the practice nurse is a 'Jack of all trades, master of none', which is a danger when considering all of the dimensions involved in the role. However, with the many skills that practice nurses possess and the development of specialist training and support, practice nurses are becoming specialists in their own right and key players within the primary healthcare team.

Table 1.2: Typical competencies of a practice nurse

a. Demonstrate an understanding of the policies and professional issues surrounding primary care and practice nursing, including an understanding of primary care trusts and Government white papers and initiatives

b. Demonstrate an understanding of the polices and professional issues within the practice, including practice protocols, policies, health and safety, confidentiality, record keeping and accountability

c. Understand the theory and knowledge of clinical skills, including:

❖ measuring blood pressure	❖ cervical smear
❖ urine testing	❖ dressings/wound care
❖ removal of sutures	❖ blood glucose monitoring
❖ ear irrigation	❖ venepuncture
❖ swabs for culture, eg. HSV, ear, wound	❖ peak flow measurements

d. Demonstrate competencies in the organisation and management of chronic disease management, including; health promotion (women's and men's health), asthma, diabetes, coronary heart disease and prevention

e. Management skills, including: organisation of treatment room and stock, assessing health needs of patients, communication skills, time management, items of service claims, developing protocols and guidelines, and understanding audit

f. An ability to develop professionally and personally, including; reflective practice, mentorship, clinical supervision, personal development planning

g. An ability to be flexible and accept change

Nurses considering a position in general practice

Practice nurses are generally employed by general practitioners who are independent contractors, running small businesses. When applying for a practice nurse post the nurse may be offered a formal interview or at least an initial meeting with the prospective employer. It is important to have planned for this and be clear about the information that will be needed, and the questions that you may need to ask about the post.

The many responsibilities and dimensions of the role are such that it makes it important for both the general practitioner and the nurse to know what care the nurse is competent to give. Many general practitioners are under the impression that general nurse training covers all aspects of nursing within general practice, this is not true.

When applying for the post it is useful to view the job description beforehand and, if available, a job specification. This will indicate the knowledge and experience required. If no experience is required or is not specified the prospective candidate needs to be sure about what training and support will be given on commencement of the post. If the practice is willing to take an inexperienced nurse, then the nurse should establish how training and support will be achieved and over what period of time.

Practice nurses are employed on various pay scales, most often, but not always, under Whitley Council terms and conditions. Hours, responsibilities and holiday allowance will differ from practice to practice and it is important to establish the terms of employment before commencing in post.

Job descriptions and contracts of employment may also differ greatly between practices, with some practice nurses not holding a job description. When applying for a job in the civil service a job description would be provided before interview, probably with the application form, so that the applicant for the post may have their skills and knowledge judged against the job criteria. It can be seen from *Table 1.2* — showing typical areas of competence needed for a practice nurse role — that even when practising at a minimum level, certain competencies are essential. Many practices expect the nurse to manage their own case load from commencement of post, often without supervision. Some practices or primary care groups may provide an induction programme, training, mentorship and clinical supervision. It is important to determine what support will be available, before accepting the post.

It will be useful to request a tour of the practice and its equipment and facilities in order to form an overall impression of the surgery. It is advisable to establish how much the practice is willing to invest in the training of staff including nurses and whether they have a policy on study leave. It is also useful to talk to other nurses within the practice, especially the current post holder.

Getting to know the practice

Once you have got the job, it is useful to build up a brief profile of the practice. This will enable the nurse to gain an insight into the resources available within the practice and plan the delivery of care needed to address the needs of the practice population. If a practice has a high population of those under twenty-four years old, the plan of care is likely to include addressing child and adolescent health, such as child immunisations, contraception and family planning. If, however, the practice population has a high percentage of elderly patients the focus of care and the provision of services is likely to be very different. Points to consider when building up a brief profile of the practice are illustrated in *Table 1.3* and ideally should be reviewed and updated at least annually.

Table 1.3: Points to consider when profiling a practice

❖ Patient population, including breakdown of ages, eg. over sixty-five years old, under five years old, sixteen to twenty-five years old

❖ The numbers for smokers, alcohol consumption, obesity and an age/sex breakdown

❖ The uptake rates for cervical smears and immunisations

❖ Role of staff, both within the practice and in the primary care team and supporting services and their qualifications and specialities

❖ Practice services and clinics already provided or needing to be developed

❖ Local services available to patients; cardiac rehabilitation, community clinics and services, eg. chiropody

❖ Profile of general practitioners within the practice and who specialises in which areas of medicine

❖ Resources available in the practice both for patient care and for staff training and development

The Red Book and the practice nurse

The Red Book, which may be dubbed the bible of general practice, was published originally in 1966 by the Minister of Health (now the Secretary of State) (Ellis *et al*, 1993). It holds information about what general practitioners need to know, including information and regulations such as those required under their terms of service of the NHS contract and how they are to be paid for those services. Most practices are required to follow *The Red Book*, apart from those that have been set up as medical services pilot schemes (PMS). These schemes were developed to explore new ways of working, which may have been constrained by the rules within *The Red Book*.

Although it is not necessary for practice nurses to know all the details within *The Red Book*, it is useful to understand the principles and how they effect their employment and training. With some practice nurses developing their role and looking towards a partnership in the practice it is even more important to understand the principles of *The Red Book*.

The Red Book includes how GPs' pay is determined (although some PMS pilots are exploring alternative ways of employing GPs such as salaried options) and how they are remunerated for their work or 'items of service'.

The Red Book also defines what practice is required to be achieved in child health surveillance (22: 1.6), minor surgery procedure (42: 1–6) and that newly registered patient health checks should be offered within twenty-eight days. Again, this is often the practice nurse's responsibility to carry out and claim for.

Guidelines are also given for the care that patients over the age of seventy-five should receive — stating that each patient should be offered a consultation and domiciliary visit to assess whether they require any medical support or treatment. Anything that appears to be affecting the patient's health should be recorded. The over seventy-five health checks are usually delegated by general practitioners to practice nurses, district nurses or health visitors.

The general practitioner's terms of service also include a requirement to submit an annual report, which should include details about how many patients are diabetic, asthmatic, overweight, smoking and consuming over the recommended limit of alcohol. Again, this may be the responsibility of the practice nurse to give guidance or carry out the audits for such a report and this should be determined at the onset of employment.

Every general practitioner and/or practice manager should have a copy of *The Red Book*, which should be included in any induction programme so that those new to practice nursing can understand its implications to their role.

Considering practice nursing as a career

> *It seems a commonly received idea among men and even among women themselves that it requires nothing but a disappointment in love, the want of an object, a general disgust or incapacity for other things, to turn a woman into a good nurse.*

Florence Nightingale, 1859

Nursing — a profession?

Since the early record of nursing in the 1800s, nursing has progressed greatly in aspiring to reach professionalism. Records show that nursing care contributed to a fall in the surgical death rate from 40% to 8% (Burdett, 1893), and this led to nursing being regarded as valuable, establishing its position in society. The progress has been slow and not without problems, but its status today is regarded by most as a profession. Due to the fact that professionalisation has been a slow, gradual process as the occupation has matured it may be that some areas of nursing are further forward than others.

Pavalko (1971) defines professionalism within a continuum, which includes many dimensions. When comparing practice nursing to the continuum it achieves most of the criteria of a profession, including autonomy: practice nurses assess, plan, deliver and evaluate the care given and, with the development of the advanced nurse practitioner, are autonomous practitioners in their own right. The role is also relevant to the social values of the public. When planning care practice nurses consider the social and cultural needs of the patient and the population, therefore practice nursing could be considered as being at the leading edge of primary care.

Training and education are fundamental to nursing and not least to practice nursing with the development of specialist practice nurse courses. Although training in the past has been *ad hoc* (Atkin and

Lunt, 1993), with the development of new roles within practice nursing, training and education has developed accordingly and many organisations who provide further education are now tailoring their courses to meet the needs of practice nurses. Practice nurses, along with fellow professionals, are regulated by codes, ethics and guidelines provided by its statutory body the UKCC (now the NMC), which again suggests that the practice nurse should be considered a professional.

Despite the fact that nursing has progressed, many critics still believe that nursing work involves little more than being a handmaiden to doctors, especially as practice nurses are still largely employed by the medical profession. The future of primary care suggests that practice nurses may be employed by other organisations, such as primary care trusts (PCTs) or set up practice on their own, either privately or as part of the Primary Care Act personal medical services (PMS) pilot schemes, and this helps practice nursing, as a profession, to become more autonomous and move further along the professional continuum. Although critics who believe that nursing is no more than a vocation of people who are primarily carers are not entirely correct, this element should not be underestimated; it is still a very valuable part of nursing and perhaps one that separates nursing from the medical profession. If the strive for professionalism undermines the caring element, this could have very bad implications for nursing, and nurses could lose the respect and the support from the public that nursing 'angels' have largely received.

The career structure is taking shape within general practice, although there are still many titles used and discrepancies regarding the scope and capabilities of various levels of nurse. The UKCC have been working with the ENB to try to define the levels and the role of nurses within general practice. The career structure emerging appears to follow the path demonstrated in *Figure 1.2* and is similar to the structure of other areas of nursing. Grades and role definitions still need to be addressed and as they continue to bemuse nurses, it is no surprise that GPs are likewise unclear as to the scope of the nurse's role.

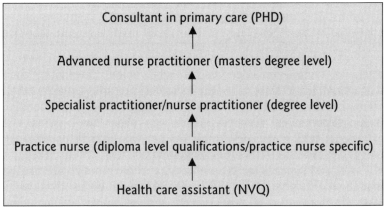

Figure 1.2: The emerging career structure in practice nursing

Consultant in primary care: This is a fairly new role first introduced by Tony Blair as part of the *NHS Plan* (DoH, 2000) and one which will link the practical side of the role with academia. The nurse will usually be required to hold a masters level degree or PhD.

Advanced nurse practitioner: An innovative and autonomous nurse who has obtained a MSc advanced nursing practice qualification. The nurse will practice at an advanced level and possess the necessary qualities to:

- assess
- investigate and manage a range of patients at an advanced level
- be a reflective practitioner who may critically appraise practice
- be an effective agent, involved in research and evidence-based practice
- examine
- be an effective leader and role model within the practice
- facilitate educational development within the clinical environment
- be an active part of a multidisciplinary team

Specialist practitioner (practice nursing): This role was set out in the UKCC's document in 1994 along with the post-registration education and practice (PREP) proposals. The UKCC said that specialist nursing practitioners were expected to demonstrate higher levels of clinical decision making and be able to monitor and improve standards of care through supervision of practice, clinical audit, developing and leading practice, contributing to research, teaching and supporting professional colleagues (UKCC, 1994).

Specialist practitioner programmes must be at first degree level and approved by the ENB. They will normally involve no less than one academic year's full-time study (RCN, 1999).

There are many practice nurses who enjoy developing their managerial, leadership, supporting and teaching role as well as their clinical role. Mentorship is expanding within general practice and many experienced practice nurses can share their skills and experience with nurses new to the field or who may be undertaking courses in order to further their development.

Clinical supervision is another area where practice nurses find that their reflective skills and leadership qualities are invaluable. With the formation of primary care groups, nurses — including practice nurses — are being represented on the primary care boards, resulting in an increased responsibility and representation in the healthcare field.

With the release of numerous strategies and documents, there are many professional opportunities open to nurses especially within primary care. As a new practice nurse, becoming clinically competent is the first step, with the second being to gain as much experience as possible. Once competent, there are many avenues open for professional development and progression including various innovations and nurse-led projects.

Practice nursing models — bio-medical *vs* nursing

This section explores the relationship between nursing theory and nursing care in practice nursing. A model is a useful way to provide a common framework in which practice nurses, along with other members of the primary healthcare team, can offer continuity of care and set high standards. As a result of developing their roles practice nurses have acquired more responsibility and because of the legal, ethical and professional aspects of the profession they must carefully reflect on the care that they plan, deliver and evaluate (Cavanagh, 1993). Kershaw and Salvage (1986) suggested that models prove useful as providing a tool that links nursing theory to practice, and help to clarify a nurse's thinking of the elements of the practice situation and their relationship with each other.

Since the introduction of the nursing process in the early 1980s, there have been many theories and models introduced both in secondary and primary care to replace the medical model often used by nurses in the past. It is important that the model chosen is appropriate both to the area of practice and to the professionals likely to be using it, otherwise it will have no valid purpose. It is also important that it does not generate more paper work while sacrificing care. There are a number of models in use and all concentrate on different methods of assessing and delivering care; the nursing models take into account the patient as a whole and they all aim to reduce ill health, restoring the patient to as normal a lifestyle as possible.

When a model is going to be used in general practice its purpose should be to clarify what the practice nurse and any others involved in the care, including relatives and carers, intend to do and to develop a minimum standard to which they will work. For a practice nurse working alone, it will be easier to decide which model to adapt to the practice, as it only needs to meet the individual's needs and criteria. Where there are other practice nurses and members of the primary healthcare team to consider, they may need to meet to discuss which model best suits their beliefs and concepts.

Some models lend themselves to practice nursing better than others. The high turnover of patients for such brief visits and the number of practices employing more than one practice nurse makes it even more necessary to work within a framework to provide consistent care.

Historically, practice nurses have worked to a medical model (concentrating on a disease or condition rather than the whole person) and there are still many who do so. Wright (1986), along with a number of nursing theorists, reported that the medical model is criticised because it places nursing as subservient to doctors' orders. Using a bio-medical model has the risk of breaking up the practice nurse's work into a series of tasks rather than dealing with the patient as a whole individual. Because the bio-medical model involves treating the disease or complaint and does not take into account any other factors or problems which the patient may have, the time normally taken by the practice nurse to assess the patient and work out a plan of care, in a nursing model, is saved. While many more patients may be seen, the benefits to the patient from the consultation may not be as effective. For instance, if they are being treated for cancer they may also be losing money because they are unable to work, which may cause hardship resulting in poor diet and living conditions, which in turn may affect their health.

When a patient is referred from the general practitioner to the practice nurse there is usually a 'complaint' or 'illness' labelling the patient, eg. Mr Smith with asthma. Although the complaint or illness is considered when assessing the patient, other influences (or stressors) experienced by the patient should be addressed. Their may be effective treatments for a teenager with asthma, but if he is reluctant to use his inhalers because of other stressors such as stigma or lack of understanding of the disease, then he may not use them. This leads to poor compliance and an exacerbation of his asthma.

Due to the many factors involved with patient care, many practice nurses have chosen to move away from the medical model and adapt the principles of nursing models instead.

The bio-medical model can be used to provide a basis for nursing care and it may be beneficial to take an eclectic approach and use the models in conjunction with one another. Cronenwett (1983) found similarities between medical and nursing models, stating that the medical model assumes that people cannot be expected to solve their own problems. Pearson *et al* (1986) argue that the knowledge base that the bio-medical model uses is objective as it results from scientific research. Nursing models and the care given within those models is far more subjective and reliant on nursing research which, in some cases, is not seen as being scientifically clear-cut. It is important for nurses when undertaking research as part of their studies to endeavour to publish those works so that the base of nursing research is increased and gains more credibility.

Among the models now used, Neuman (cited by Pearson and Vaughan, 1986) lends itself well to practice nursing. The author of the model has moved away from the bio-medical model which concentrates on treatment of illness toward a model that promotes total patient care. With the introduction of primary healthcare teams and integrated working this model lends itself well as it offers an inter-disciplinary approach and draws together the goals of all disciplines involved in health care.

Neuman includes several theories within her model, such as systems theory and stress adaptation. The person is viewed as a whole person, not just a medical condition. The model takes into account social, psychological and cultural needs and considers the way that a person interacts within his or her community or surroundings. Neuman stated that, 'intervention can begin at any point at which a stressor is either suspected or identified.' This can include preventative care as well as treatment. As a great deal of the practice nurse's role is involved with health promotion and prevention of illness this would seem to suggest the model's suitability to general practice. When assessing the patient, Neuman suggests the use of six basic questions (*Table 1.4*). When adapted to a situation in practice, eg. asking those questions of a mother with an eleven-year-old son suffering from asthma, the answers may be similar to those on the right of the table.

Table 1.4: Six basic questions

1. What do you consider to be your major problem, difficulty or concern?	1. At the moment my major area of concern is his move to secondary school. Will he be disadvantaged in any way, eg. games. Will other children taunt him for having to use his inhalers?
2. How has this affected your usual pattern of living or lifestyle?	2. He is getting very nervous about going to senior school and this seems to be making him moody and withdrawn towards us
3. Have you ever experienced a similar problem previously? If so, what was the problem and how did you handle it? Was your handling of the problem successful?	3. He has always been OK in primary school as some of his friends also have asthma. Because he is in the same classroom all of the time he can hide his inhaler and spacer in the desk
4. What do you anticipate for yourself in the future as a consequence of the present situation?	4. I am worried that this will result in him not using his inhalers and having an acute episode of his asthma
5. What are you doing and what can you do to help yourself?	5. As a family we can encourage him to take his medication and offer support. We can contact the senior school and discuss the situation with them, we have also come to the surgery to explore other sorts of inhaler devices that may be a little more discreet
6. What do you expect care givers, family, friends and others to do for you?	6. Once he has made new friends at school we can help to educate them in what asthma is, and also encourage teachers to educate the rest of the school regarding asthma

Neuman, cited by Pearson and Vaughan (1986)

The above questions and answers help a practice nurse to define the problems experienced by the patient or the patient's mother. The health needs of this young man result from the stigma and the practicalities surrounding the management of his asthma, rather than the effects of the disease itself. Nevertheless, for the boy to maintain good health these issues would need to be addressed.

Conclusion

This chapter demonstrates the importance of the decision to enter general practice and that it is an area of primary care nursing that should not be underestimated.

It is one of the very few areas of nursing where there is a single employer (the general practitioner) rather than an authority, making it even more important to ensure that the job is supported by good employment practice before making the decision to take up the post.

Once employed by the general practitioner, there should be many opportunities for increased autonomy, decision making and professional and personal development, and it is imperative that the nurse entering general practice can cope with and take advantage of this.

2

Training and support in general practice

Introduction

The changing environment of general practice and primary care means that the way we practice and the demands of our practice are always changing. With the introduction of the Government White Paper, *The new NHS — modern, dependable* (DoH, 1997), which resulted in the development of primary care groups, it is vital for practice nurses to acquire knowledge and competencies to cope with the new demands and changes. This chapter gives some principles and suggestions on how nurses new to general practice may meet the educational and training requirements to gain the skills needed for the demands of the changing and evolving role, and become and remain competent practitioners

Induction

It has been apparent from research (Atkin and Lunt, 1993) that induction and training for practice nurses has been *ad hoc*, especially when introducing a nurse from the acute sector into general practice. They also discovered in their subsequent research (Atkin and Lunt, 1995) that many general practitioners think that nurses can automatically acquire the necessary skills needed to become a practice nurse as a result of general nurse training.

This first national consensus of practice nurses in England and Wales showed that many practice nurses expressed a need for training; fewer than half had attended a formal induction and the same number had never attended a course at all. It was surprising to find that in 1998, within the Black Country, only 14% of practice nurses had received a formal induction course (Bradley, 1998) despite recommendations for induction to take place as a result of this report.

There is not one appropriate model of induction for every nurse entering general practice, but the evidence shows that implementation of an induction programme is important to nurses (Bradley, 1998). It is also apparent that the induction package and length of time for the induction period depends on the nurse's previous roles and responsibilities and needs to be flexible and tailored to suit the individual. The aim of an induction programme should be to achieve a competent practice nurse in the most effective way.

There are a number of ways to deliver an induction programme for practice nurses (*Table 2.1*). Most of these include providing the facilitation and support needed by nurses new to general practice through mentorship — a relationship between a new nurse and a mentor in which the nurse is supported, challenged and encouraged to develop in her role by the mentor.

The theoretical framework (*Figure 2.1*) shows a number of factors that contribute to the way that a practice nurse becomes competent. This suggests that the induction programme should include input from the practice, mentor, primary healthcare team and PCT and be supported by training institutions (formal courses) and literature (eg. induction pack developed by the practice).

Table 2.1: Ways to deliver an induction package
❖ In-house with nurse mentor from within the practice
❖ In-house with nurse mentor from outside the practice
❖ In-house with another member of the primary healthcare team as mentor
❖ In-house by GP
❖ In-house with induction package developed by practice — no mentor
❖ Outside practice — in mentor's practice
❖ Formal induction course with/ without mentor

There may be local guidelines for how long an induction period should last in order for those who fund it to plan resources. However, due to the variation in roles and the differing experience of nurses entering general practice, some nurses may require longer induction periods than others. This needs to be negotiated between nurse, mentor, practice and PCG. As a guide, six months would usually be considered the minimum time needed for the induction period.

Once the new practice nurse has been assigned a mentor, usually by a co-ordinator from the primary care group facilitator responsible for training or by the mentor group itself, it is useful for them to meet with the new practice nurse to negotiate a programme for the induction period. To do this, a number of factors should be considered (*Table 2.2*).

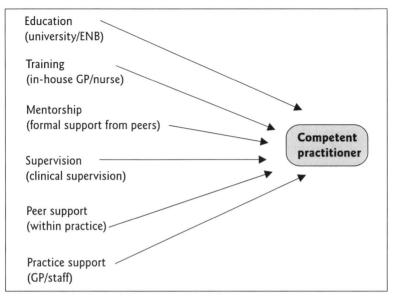

Figure 2.1: Theoretical framework for induction

Table 2.2: Factors to consider when planning induction

❖ Experience of the nurse new to general practice

❖ Job description — may be used to decide what the nurse is expected to be competent in following induction

❖ Practice agenda — it is useful to know how practice nursing fits into the practice agenda

❖ Personal agenda — the expectations of the practice nurse from the role

❖ Local agenda — are there any expectations which the primary care group have from the post (especially if they are funding the post and/or the nurse is going to be part of a pilot scheme)?

❖ National agenda — consider Government plans and strategies which may affect the care to be given, eg. *Our Healthier Nation* (DoH, 1997)

Once the competencies needed for the post have been established, a time scale and arrangements for how often the mentor and mentee will meet can be agreed. The mentee will probably require more support in the initial period of the post, meeting perhaps regularly once or twice a week, depending on circumstances.

When they meet the list of competencies can provide a basis for reflection and discussion, providing structure to the session. The mentor can work through them until both the nurse new to practice and the mentor feel confident that all competencies have been achieved.

In addition, an induction pack may prove a useful resource for the new practice nurse (*Table 2.3* shows an example of useful information). This may include information to be used on the first day of starting a post. There is nothing worse than turning up on the first day of work and not knowing who people are, or where to find the ladies room! The pack may already hold information, such as useful telephone numbers, maps of the local area or, alternatively, those pages can be left blank so that the new nurse fills them in for herself, providing a learning exercise.

Table 2.3: Information to include in an induction pack

❖ Professional details of new practice nurse, eg. PIN number (NMC), name of general practice, commencement date, professional qualifications, date of commencement in post

❖ Names and position of staff working in and attached to the practice

❖ Important contact telephone numbers or fax numbers, eg. pharmacy, district nurses, primary care group etc

❖ Layout of the surgery and location of emergency drugs, resuscitation equipment, fire extinguishers etc

❖ Map of the surrounding area of the practice showing, for example, chemist, schools, housing estates

❖ Competencies to work through with mentor

It may be difficult to know when to end the mentor/mentee relationship but once the mentor and mentee feel satisfied that the nurse new to general practice is a competent practitioner, the induction programme may be considered over and a success. The mentor should encourage the nurse to be as autonomous as possible; it is useful to keep a telephone number to contact the mentor in case she needs further help or advice.

Mentoring

The term mentor is defined by the Collins *Concise English Dictionary* (1992) as, 'wise, trusted advisor, guide' and has developed over the last few years, into a useful if not 'in vogue' tool for many professions and businesses, including nursing. A mentor has been described as, 'giving support, a role model, facilitator to learning, supervisor and assessor'.

In general practice, this is likely to be between an experienced practice nurse who has undergone training to become a mentor (although there is no standard for mentor training and this can be *ad hoc* throughout the country) and another practice nurse, usually new to general practice. Mentors may be used in other situations as can be seen in *Figure 2.2*.

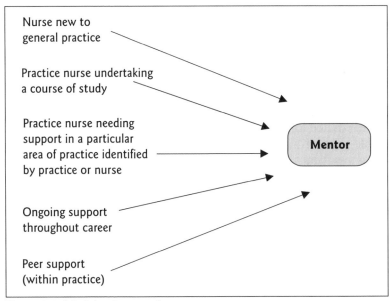

Figure 2.2: Models of mentoring

The relationship will be one where the two individuals will have the opportunity to relate with each other, where the mentor facilitates learning and allows the mentee to perform their role more effectively and so develop professionally and competently. The mentor plays a vital role in the induction period of a nurse new to general practice. The process of mentoring is especially valuable for practice nursing as many practitioners work in isolation from one another and rely on a support network for induction and professional development. The relationship between mentor and mentee may function in a formal or informal manner, it may be a system that is arranged by the employer, the health authority/PCG or arranged between practice nurses themselves. The mentor should be there to support the mentee through a number of skills gained through experience and training. The helper functions of mentoring have been defined as follows:

- adviser
- coach
- counsellor
- guide/networker
- role model
- sponsor
- teacher
- resource facilitator (Morton-Cooper *et al*, 1999).

Usually the relationship within the general practice setting is between two practice nurses. On occasions, the logistics of this may be difficult due to clashing working hours, geographical placement etc and it may be more appropriate for other professionals to mentor. The various models that may be adapted for the mentoring process are illustrated in *Figure 2.3*. Although it probably makes for a more stable relationship to have just one mentor there is no reason why other members of the team cannot contribute to the induction process by offering training and support.

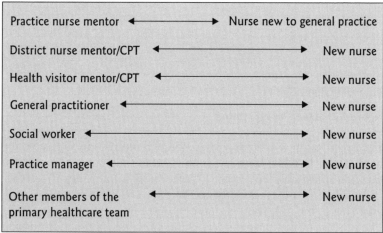

Figure 2.3: The models for mentoring

Some of the models shown may be seen to be controversial as it could be argued that nurses, other than those working in general practice, do not have the experience within that field. It is likely that all groups will have skills in mentoring, as it is a process used within most disciplines, but if experience within the field of the mentee is considered an important aspect of mentoring, other disciplines may lose credibility. The professionals identified as possible mentors, however, may form a useful part of the induction programme and it is worth exploring how inter-professional working can be included when planning an induction package.

The experienced mentor will be a continual source for advice, either face-to-face or over the telephone. In the context of the induction programme, this advice covers handling situations within the practice, such as employment issues, career pathways as well as clinical advice.

During the induction period the mentor will also act as coach, helping the mentee to set objectives and goals and providing constructive feedback. The extent of the mentor's knowledge of the geographical area and the area of practice nursing means that they will be an excellent guide, introducing the mentor to people, groups and places where they may obtain the experience they need. The mentor must be careful not to take on the tasks themselves, but encourage the mentee to make their own contacts and arrange meetings, making it a learning experience.

The relationship may be for a set period agreed between the practice and the mentor. However, many mentors remain in contact with the mentee and continue to be a source of support and knowledge throughout their career in general practice.

Clinical supervision

Clinical supervision was a concept from the Government's document *A Vision for the Future* (DoH, 1993) which defined and recommended the implementation of clinical supervision. It too plays an important part in practice nursing, especially for nurses new to general practice. It is a term used to describe a formal process of professional support and learning which enables practice nurses, as well as other healthcare professionals, to develop knowledge, confidence and competence and realise the importance of taking responsibility for their own practice.

Clinical supervision has been widely discussed in nursing literature and has many definitions and interpretations. Butterworth and Faugier (1992), probably the pioneers of the introduction of clinical supervision, define it as, 'an interactive process between providers of health care, which enables the development of professional knowledge and skills'. The definition is clear about the expected outcome of clinical supervision but does not suggest how the process works or, indeed, which professionals should be involved.

In 1995, the UKCC issued a position statement on clinical supervision which avoided being prescriptive, providing only principles to be interpreted and implemented in a flexible way to suit the individual situation. In general practice, for instance, it would be impossible to duplicate the model used in the hospital setting due to the logistics of practice nursing hours, employment and places of work. The UKCC therefore gave an opportunity for the various disciplines including practice nurses to develop a model of their own.

Many nurses and critics felt threatened by the implementation of supervision and some felt that it had managerial overtones.

The development of primary care is the main focus of the Government's White Paper, *The new NHS — modern, dependable* (DoH, 1997). It debates that for primary care to function effectively there is an urgent need to develop and implement a process of clinical supervision. Clinical supervision has yet to prove that it is, indeed, efficient in achieving the objectives for which it has been developed (*Table 2.4*) as these can be difficult to measure.

Table 2.4: Objectives of clinical supervision
❖ Enhancing patient care
❖ Encouraging professional growth
❖ Promoting self-assurance and confidence
❖ Reducing sickness and absence rates

Clinical supervisors within general practice will normally be selected at primary care group level. It is important that they hold the skills needed to supervise and receive comprehensive training for the role. The role of supervisor and the skills needed are closely linked to those of a mentor, however, supervisors need to be able to understand the function and process of clinical supervision. The role of supervisor has been defined as:

> *A professional practitioner who provides an interactive, professional partnership where there is shared responsibility for stimulating critical reflection, reviewing and assessing personal performance, as well as providing support and emotional refreshment.*

> Morton-Cooper *et al*, 1999

There are a number of different models of clinical supervision used in primary care to date and some have been more successful than others (*Figure 2.4*). The difficulty with providing support for practice nurses is that they are usually working in isolation and due to time restraints it is difficult to hold regular clinical supervision meetings. The models used in practice nursing tend to be those using a network of supervisors.

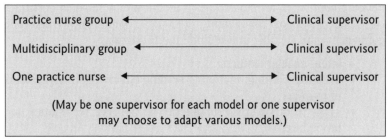

Figure 2.4: Models of practice nurse clinical supervision

Supervision can provide a protected forum to enable practice nurses, especially those new to general practice, to gain support and confidence from qualified supervisors and benefit from their experience. If there is an accommodation for supervision it will provide another form of support for nurses new to general practice.

Many practice nurses choose to be supervisors, using their knowledge, experience and expertise to help other nurses. Nurses new to general practice benefit from undertaking clinical supervision for the reasons discussed and it may be the norm, in future, for general practitioners to accommodate this within the contract of employment. However, because the benefits of supervision are difficult to measure in terms of improved patient care and cost effectiveness, it may take time for healthcare professionals and general practitioners to be convinced.

A typical supervision session involves discussion and analysis of a critical incident chosen by supervisor or supervisee, a patient case study chosen by either, or any area causing concern to either supervisor or supervisee.

Training and PREP

The UKCC (1994) recognised that nursing is evolving and recommended lifelong learning with post-registration education and practice (PREP) to ensure that the best possible care would be given to patients and clients. The UKCC stated that PREP would help keep nurses up-to-date with new developments in practice and encourage them to think and reflect (UKCC, 2001), and made a ruling that every registered nurse is required to undertake the equivalent of a minimum of five days study every three years. They would also be required, if requested, to present the details of their education and professional development when re-registering, in the form of a personal portfolio.

The ways of maintaining and developing knowledge and competence are flexible and include the following:

- attendance at lectures
- distance learning, including reading educational supplements in journals
- visits to other areas of practice to observe techniques and procedures
- personal research, ie. undertaking a literature search in a library.

PREP relies on self-appraisal, however, it must be stressed that the type of study undertaken should be relevant to the practice nurse's role and professional registration. Recognising that some nurses may have difficulty in defining the areas in which they need to be competent, the UKCC also established five broad categories related to the nursing role to help nurses plan areas of study. These are:

- patient, client and colleague support
- care enhancement
- practice development
- reducing risk
- education development.

For nurses new to general practice there may be many areas in which competencies need to be achieved. It is appropriate to discuss and prioritise those areas with a mentor. The evidence documented as part of an induction programme may be used for PREP and should be included in their portfolio.

Personal development plans

Personal development plans are as simple or as complicated as needed. The practice or primary care group in which the nurse is working may already have a proforma or guideline developed. An example of a personal development plan is demonstrated in *Figure 2.5*.

Where am I now?

A record of the qualifications and study completed.		
Date	**Study**	**Qualification**
1.3.82	General nurse training	RGN
1.5.93	Asthma	Dip Asthma

Clinical responsibilities (circle)

	Level of involvement		
Asthma	min	intermediate	max
Diabetes	min	intermediate	max
Congenital heart disease (CHD)	min	intermediate	max
Cervical cytology	min	intermediate	max
Family planning	min	intermediate	max

Minimum involvement usually means that the practice nurse carries out initial checks or tasks but does not take overall responsibility for the care of the patient.

Intermediate involvement usually means that the practice nurse plans and carries out most of the care of the patient but the clinic/session is always supported by the general practitioner or other practice nurses.

Maximum care usually indicates that the practice nurse plans, delivers and takes responsibility for the patient/clinic with little or no involvement from the general practitioner.

Now identify the legislative needs of the practice/primary care group

Health and safety

First Aid

etc

Courses needed
1 CPR update
2
3

Now identify any additional skills/clinics which may develop in the next three years

Clinic/skills	**Expected date**	**Study/training needed**
Women's health	Sept 2001	Cervical smear update

Now consider where you would like to be professionally

Advanced nurse practitioner

Nurse practitioner/specialist practitioner

Clinical supervisor

Mentor

Trainer

Higher grade

Now prioritise those needs and fill in the plan below

Qualification/skills required	Details of training/ course available	Date to achieve	Date completed

Figure 2.5: A personal development plan

Developing skills and competencies in line with the challenging world of primary care is the key to improving the delivery and quality of care to the public and is recommended both by the UKCC (1994) in line with PREP, and as part of the implementation of clinical governance (a recent concept introduced by the government to improve high standards of care by a number of activities, see *Chapter 4*). The Chief Medical Officer (CMO) has stated that all practices should have a practice development plan to which individual healthcare professionals contribute with their personal development plans (Gallen, 2000).

The aim of personal development planning in general practice nursing is to identify future training needs and set objectives for the following twelve months as part of the appraisal and IPR scheme. This will not only enable the practice to plan both time and resources needed as part of their practice development plan, but if fed back to the primary care group, it could assist in the future planning and funding for training.

Personal development planning is about viewing the professional development needs of staff in a more structured way, while considering the needs of the practice, profession and personal needs. When planning future development, a new practice nurse should examine the best ways of achieving skills, while considering the resources of the practice. Practice nurses also need to think about how much of their own time they are prepared to spend in achieving their individual aims.

Once the training and areas of professional development have been identified, it is important to prepare a proposal for whoever is likely to be funding the course and/or providing time out of the practice. The practice manager may be a valuable resource to help the practice nurse put this together.

Approval should be sought from whoever holds the responsibility for approving study or study leave, eg. practice nurse manager, practice manager or general practitioner. In order to do this, take a few minutes to prepare the plan and the supporting case. The objectives once identified from the plan need to be prioritised. This is important as the very nature of general practice means that the practice nurse may not be able to leave the practice for long periods of time for study.

It is also worth considering the priorities of whoever approves the request and how your request will be viewed. If there is a practice policy for study leave this should also be considered. It may be useful to include in the request the estimated cost of the training, the method of training (eg. in-house, courses, personal study, long distance) and examine staffing levels and possible locum costs at the time of any course.

When requesting study leave, an explanation of how the knowledge will be used, the benefits to patient care and how the knowledge can be shared with others within the practice or wider primary care group may serve to strengthen the request. If any assignments are expected as part of a course, then their subject should be useful to the practice as well as the practitioner. When requesting study leave or funding, the benefits in terms of patient care should be emphasised.

Reflective practice

Providing high quality care to patients involves not only identifying and updating training needs but practising as a reflective practitioner.

The principles used within reflective practice are not new. We reflect on issues and events in our lives every day. For example, when taking a cake out of the oven — if it is soggy, flat or tasteless we may reflect on why that has happened and next time try adding some more baking powder, altering the oven temperature or buy a cake from the local shop instead! In nursing we cannot always afford to try something else next time to see if it works, especially if it affects patient care. Reflection in nursing needs to be a more structured process so that we analyse what has happened and explore how the situation may be handled differently next time it occurs. The best way to do this is by using a reflective model or framework. There are a number of models that have been developed, all of which lend themselves to situations differently.

When entering general practice the nurse may already have some knowledge and experience regarding reflective practice, as it is a concept which is integrated into most areas of nursing and a large part of the nurse training programmes.

It is useful to understand how these skills may be utilised as part of the new role in general practice, as the logistics may differ slightly from an alternative setting. Reflective practice can form a useful part of the induction process for nurses new to general practice, helping to consolidate the training in the first few months as well as being used within clinical supervision sessions, allowing the nurse to become more perceptive to practice.

Reflection or reflective practice has a number of definitions: the word reflection originates from the verb *Reflectere*, to bend or turn backwards. It has been defined as:

> *The process of internally examining and exploring an issue of concern, triggered by an experience, which creates and clarifies meaning in terms of self, and which results in a changed conceptual perspective.*

Boyd and Fales, 1983

Reflection could be considered as examining an incident or situation in a new way using different perspectives. The following is an example of the type of incident that could be used to reflect upon:

> Patient A enters the nurse's room for a vaccination for tetanus, the patient appears agitated and is quite rude to the new practice nurse. The nurse attempts to give information about the follow-up and side-effects of the vaccine, despite the rude response. The patient receives the vaccine and leaves the room.

During this incident the nurse may have felt uncomfortable and slightly threatened by the situation, but incidents that have been a 'success', leaving the nurse feeling that it was handled well may also be used for reflection.

Most incidents may be examined from various angles, including the nurse's, the patient's and even reception staff. The nurse may have felt uncomfortable and slightly annoyed, but there may have been a good reason why the patient acted in that manner. The patient may have been nervous through not knowing the new nurse, she may even have been annoyed if she had been kept waiting a long time for her appointment. There may have been a member of reception staff who was unaware that the patient was waiting.

There are a number of different reflective models found in literature which may be used to reflect on this situation.

As many practice nurses work in isolation, they need to use reflective practice on their own, using one of the various models, eg. Atkins and Murphy (1994), Johns (1994) and Gibbs (1988) being the most common.

Figure 2.6 demonstrates how reflective practice may be carried out in primary care.

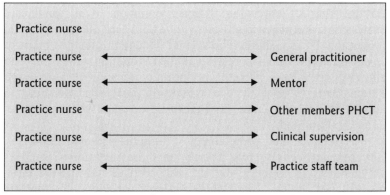

Figure 2.6: Carrying out reflective practice in general practice — with whom?

A reflective diary, log or journal may be useful to document critical incidents as they occur so that they are not forgotten and can be reflected upon later. These are also useful to take to a clinical supervision meeting as critical incident examples.

Multidisciplinary training

Traditionally, training in health care has been delivered separately to individual professional groups. Nursing students and medical students' paths do not often cross except for occasional instances on the wards. Similarly, inter-professional training has not been very common. In the past, school nurses, district nurses, health visitors and practice nurses have, in most instances, been trained separately. Reeves (2000) suggested that poor communication and collaboration between medics and nursing staff may be a result of fragmented training programmes.

In order to equip health professionals to improve ill health and reduce health inequalities the Government has recommended, in at least two of its documents (the *NHS Plan* and *A health service of all the talents: developing the NHS workforce*, DoH, 2000) that changes should take place in the educational arena. The *NHS Plan* recommends that joint training across professions should take place, especially in common core areas such as communication skills and the structure and principles of the NHS. This may result in a very different approach to practice nurse training and induction in the future.

The Government recognises in the *NHS Plan* that there are

certain areas of education that are common to all healthcare professions, and states that these will be delivered jointly across the professions in the future. The second document includes plans to develop a new common core programme for training professionals to allow students and staff the opportunity to switch careers and training paths more easily. This may result in significant changes to nurse training and open the door for nurses to take fast access routes to medical training.

To deliver this programme of training and education, the Government needs to rely heavily on those institutions, such as universities and colleges, that are able to plan and provide these programmes. Finch (2000) holds reservations and states that the universities and colleges require greater clarity about the objectives of the health service and what is defined by inter-professional and multidisciplinary training.

In some areas multi-professional training is already taking place. Seabrook (1998), reporting on a study of nurses used to teach junior doctors, found that nurses teaching doctors helped to break down the barrier between doctors and nurses.

This may affect nurses new to general practice in the future as they may well receive an induction training package not only from members of their own profession but from others, eg. social services, school nurses, doctors and primary care group members, including the public. The advantages and disadvantages to practice nurses are:

Advantages

❖ A breakdown of barriers between professions.

❖ An opportunity to learn about other professionals and their role.

❖ It will help to provide a more seamless service — all singing from the same hymn sheet.

❖ Practice nurse roles will be better understood by other professionals.

Disadvantages

❖ Diluted training (trying to meet everyone's needs within the group).

❖ Training arranged by other professionals for practice nurses may not be appropriate.

The Government is hoping that training institutions may act as a catalyst for breaking down the professional barriers to promote more effective working.

Conclusion

Dedicating a chapter to induction, training and education for the nurse new to general practice, highlights the importance that this plays in her role. To ensure that a practitioner is competent and able to undertake her own caseload and provide a high quality service to patients as soon as possible after commencing relies solely on the quality of training and support received in the first vital months.

3

Primary care and the new practice nurse

Introduction

The introduction of changes through the Government's strategies and policies has had many implications for nursing as a profession, not least practice nurses.

For practice nursing to be among those at the leading edge of primary care, they need to be aware of these changes and to be involved in any further consultation processes when new papers are being developed. This will enable practice nurses to manage the changes and not merely survive them.

This chapter explains the implications that the Government's White Paper, *The new NHS — modern, dependable* (DoH, 1997) is having on practice nursing itself, namely the formation in the past of primary care groups (PCGs) and now primary care trusts (PCTs), as well as the effects of other major government documents.

A whistle-stop tour of PCGs and PCTs

Primary care groups and primary care trusts formed as a result of the Government White Paper, *The new NHS — modern, dependable* (DoH, 1997). The Government wanted to develop the primary care group to be more perceptive to the needs of the local community than the health authority, while delivering more appropriate care sensitive to the needs of the locality.

The three main functions of the PCGs are:

❖ To improve the health and address health inequalities of their community.

❖ To develop primary care and community services.

❖ To commission a range of hospital services which meet their patients' needs.

NHS Executive, 1997

Many primary care groups were born from existing general practitioner commissioning groups and started at various levels according to skills and experience (*Table 3.1*). In the first instance, they were all committees of the relevant health authority (NHS, 1999), but since legislation to enable them to evolve into primary care trusts has been passed this has all changed.

Table 3.1: Levels of PCGs

Level 1:	Functions as an advisory sub-committee of the health authority on commissioning matters
Level 2:	Operates as a sub-committee of the health authority, with devolved responsibility for the commissioning, budget and primary care development in line with population need
Level 3:	Become established as freestanding bodies accountable to health authorities for commissioning care
Level 4:	Become established as freestanding bodies accountable to health authorities for commissioning care and with added responsibility for the provision of community services for their population

The government issued guidelines for how they expected the groups to form, the boundaries and the average number of patients to be served by the PCG. There were many issues involved such as into whose boundary the PCG would fall? Social services and other community services often worked within different boundaries than the general practitioners.

Each primary care group had a primary care board, made up of a representative group of primary care professionals and lay people (*Table 3.2*). They were appointed for periods of three years or less. There were various ways of electing these representatives but mostly it was done by the professionals' and lay people's representatives.

This change meant that the role of the health authority also changed from being at the forefront of commissioning, rationing and the organisation of primary care, to one of facilitation for the developing PCGs.

The change over to primary care groups has had implications for practice nurses. It has provided the first opportunity for nurses to be represented by themselves rather than by general practitioners, as was often the case before. Although most general practitioners retain their independent status, all practices are obliged to belong to a primary care group. This means that the practice has to be accountable to the group, work collaboratively and share information and practice. There are a number of requirements through clinical governance for practices to provide high quality, appropriate care in line with their colleagues and other practices.

Many primary care groups have converted to primary care trusts (PCTs) and a total of forty trusts operate in England at the present time, with the rest of the PCGs planning to become trusts by 2004. Primary care trusts are freestanding, statutory bodies with greater flexibility and freedom, responsible for delivering better care to the population (NHS Executive, 1999).

As employment arrangements for general practitioners change (some general practitioners are being employed by trusts), some practice nurses may find themselves being employed by trusts in the future, which means that employment arrangements, scales and role definitions may change; others fear that this will challenge their influence on grades and working arrangements (Radford, 2000). For those practice nurses who work under poor employment practice (such as those who have not received a contract or GPs who have failed to honour the recommended practice nurses' pay rises) it may be beneficial. Change brings with it opportunities and practice nurses need to make sure that they hold a high profile within the PCTs, as they have strived to do within the PCGs, so that their needs are heard and addressed.

Table 3.2: Configuration of the primary care group board

Four to seven general practitioners

One to two community nurses (practice nurses, health visitors, district nurses) — may be decided by a ballot of nurses or by appointment through the health authority. Some areas may opt for nursing forums to choose candidates

One social service officer nominee

One lay member

One health authority non-executive

One primary care group chief officer, employed by the health authority, appointed by the primary care group board and accountable to the group chairman. The chief officer is responsible for managing the primary care group, but the chairman takes ultimate responsibility

Primary healthcare teams

There is not one definition for a primary healthcare team, although it is generally accepted that the primary healthcare team consists of all professionals who contribute to the care of the patient in the community. This includes professionals such as chiropodists, physiotherapists, and dieticians who often practice from within GPs' surgeries and share a mutual interest in improving health. Key themes that are shared have been defined within the Government's document, *Shared contributions, Shared benefits* (DoH, 1997c), as;

- an approach which is multidisciplinary and generalist
- a concern with health and the whole person
- a concern for people which is not confined to their status as patients
- a concern for groups of people (for public health), often a geographical population, for general practice, for most purposes the practice list
- an ongoing relationship with the individuals and/or communities, often over a number of years
- an interest in prevention, early diagnosis, treatment and care across the whole spectrum of diseases
- responsiveness to the views of patients, carers and others, and an awareness of community.

It is important that the primary healthcare team (PHCT) is able to meet on a regular basis to discuss and plan health care. This may be difficult due to the working patterns of the individuals within the primary healthcare team and the availability of time out for meetings.

The function of primary care teams is to take a more pro-active role in responding to the health needs of their population and the practice nurse plays an important role in this. The practice nurse, along with the rest of the primary healthcare team, are best placed to recognise the needs of the population and to tailor their services accordingly. They may deal, for instance, with many people with smoking-related diseases and, as part of the PHCT, they can assess to what extent smoking is a problem and form a strategy which meets local need to address the problem.

For a primary healthcare team to function effectively there should be a protocol or agreement between members to define their roles and responsibilities. It is also a good idea to come to an agreement on how often the team will meet and what the objectives of the primary healthcare team will be.

To be effective, the members of the team need to have a good working relationship with each other and understand that each member of the team is likely to have a different strength. Plant (1987) suggests that these strengths will encompass any or all of the following:

- experience
- technical training
- special skills
- some unique contribution.

It would be useful to map and analyse those strengths when the team first meet, so that those strengths may be employed within the team resulting in higher personal satisfaction among the members.

The concept of integrated teams may bring negative responses as nurses may have a fear of change and be under the misconception that integration means 'Jack-of-all-trades and master of none' as the role boundaries erode. This should not be the case: roles within the team should be enhanced and valued as a result of better communication and understanding of everyone else's role.

There may be a breakdown of traditional roles and working practices needed within the team and this may not be accepted as readily by some professions or purchasers.

The practice nurse role has extended to include considerable health promotion and it has been argued that this has resulted in an erosion of the health visiting role.

Galvin, 1999

Some health visitors have been reported as feeling threatened and undervalued in the PHCT (Wade, 1995). It could be argued that district nurses are feeling the same although the overlap between their role and others within the team may be smaller.

Within a PHCT there are a great many professionals working with the same aim: to provide a cost effective, high class service, delivered by the appropriate people to the population. It may be beneficial for a nurse new to general practice to shadow each member of the team to learn about their roles and how they can be integrated with each other. Integration is about different professionals, eg. district nurses, health visitors, school nurses etc bringing together their skills and knowledge so that the needs of the population are met, and duplications or gaps within the service are identified and solved. The Government's recent strategies and policies, including the *NHS Plan* (DoH, 2000), state that nurses should work with other agencies which implies an extension of the primary healthcare team to include agencies such as social services, local councils, and schools.

The rationale behind the introduction of integrated nursing teams in primary care was to improve the quality and access of services for patients and create a change in culture where professionals share problems, decisions and achievements. The integrated nursing team would develop services in response to the needs of the local population and may even reduce management costs, allowing more resources to be used for patient care.

Belonging to an integrated nursing team should lead to an increase in autonomy and nurse-led initiatives. The team does not have to rely on the various employers to 'sanction' developments or 'ask' their employer's permission to go ahead with initiatives. Nurses are well placed to identify the needs of the nursing team and the population whom they serve and, with the differing skills within the team, they should be able to commission new developments and services. Integration also provides a flexibility across role boundaries, for example, a practice nurse who is unable to see her over-75s who are housebound, may liaise with the health visitor and district nurse, so that if the patient is already receiving care from those services the over-75s check may be incorporated within their next visit. This will avoid duplicating visits and also ensure that all the over-75s receive a visit or invitation for a health check. The practice nurse may have a high incidence of school age children on her asthma register, and may find it useful to liaise with the school nurse for education and monitoring of these children.

To operate effectively as an integrated team, the team will have meetings and this again may put pressure on its members who have a large caseload. Differing employers and times of work may also pose a barrier to meetings. The problems of meeting and working together as a PHCT are highlighted in a number of studies. Hart (1996) found that considerable effort is needed to maintain the PHCT as an active group, due to other commitments of the PHCT's individual members or differing employers or working times. One of the benefits of practice nurses being employed by a trust instead of an individual GP, is that it might make it easier to meet with other members of the trust and to agree common objectives.

The primary healthcare team needs to have a common goal or perspective and work together to achieve this. If individuals within the team are pulling in different directions with different goals then the final aim may not be achieved. The team needs to be respondent to user needs while considering the needs of the primary healthcare team, local agenda and national agenda, especially in public health issues.

In the past, practice nurses were predominantly involved in 'treating patients' using a medical model and an individualist approach. Following the publication of the Government's *Health of the Nation* (DoH, 1986) and subsequently, since *Saving Lives: Our*

Healthier Nation (DoH, 1997b) there has been a paradigm shift towards a culture of health promotion and preventative nursing care (public health). This involves practice nurses as well as other health professionals, especially since the development of primary health-care teams. Therefore, it is important to examine the role of the practice nurse within the public health domain.

Public health and the practice nurse

Before the role of the practice nurse can be evaluated or examined as part of the public health domain, it is important to understand the definition of public health and how it fits into primary care. Public health can be defined as:

> *The knowledge, skills and attitudes that together are applied to developing an understanding of the public's health and trying to improve it.*

O'Brien, 1996

It is a method of examining the health and the causes of ill health within a whole community, rather than treating each patient individually.

Ashton *et al* (1990) gave the analogy:

> *A life saver standing alongside a fast flowing river was continuously fishing drowning people out of a river and resuscitating them. The life saver was so busy and involved in this activity that he had no time to walk upstream to find out why so many people were falling into the river.*

The public health domain requires practice nurses to examine health at a much wider level than the practice boundary, to discover the causes of health problems in society as a whole and to try to build strategies to overcome them. For instance, a practice nurse who has time constraints may be treating several patients for diseases caused through smoking but not have time to carry out smoking cessation clinics. If the problem was examined through the primary care team or a primary care group using critical incident analysis (gathering and analysing data from many practices) it may emerge that other practices were having the same problem. It may then be decided that those patients and many more would benefit from a district-wide policy to combat smoking, eg. community smoking cessation clinics, preventing people from smoking in public buildings, places of work, etc.

The desire for public health initiatives was expressed in the World Health Organization's global strategy of health for all by the year 2000 (WHO, 1978). This recommended that primary care be the centre to the attainment of this goal. The organisation also recognised that the strategy would depend on the collaboration between different sectors and agencies.

As public health involves the health of the whole community all those who serve the community need to be considered. If members of the primary healthcare team, social services, police, etc. worked only within their own disciplines the service becomes fragmented, leading to initiatives and care packages being duplicated or not delivered at all. This is one of the reasons for the development of the PCGs to encourage multi-agency co-operation and collaboration.

Since the introduction of the health service reforms (DoH, 1990), the Government has expected health care to be based on health needs. Health needs assessment is now a prime responsibility of the primary healthcare team, including practice nurses (Hutchby, 1996). The public healthcare needs of the population differ in each area and the PCG's function is to commission health care as near to the patient as possible. Services should reflect the demographic and social needs of the area that professionals serve. Practice nurses, along with other professionals, should use practice information regarding morbidity, age, sex registers and audits to help compile practice or community profiles (as demonstrated in *Chapter 1*).

Epidemiology is another important aspect of public health in which the practice nurse may require some knowledge. Epidemiology can be defined as:

> *The study of the distribution and the determinants of health-related states or events in specified populations and the application of this study to the control of health problems.*

Last, 1988

It is important that practice nurses gain a knowledge of epidemiology to understand why tasks are being done. Screening in general practice relies heavily on epidemiology to provide the evidence that the care being planned, delivered and evaluated is appropriate to the population.

After the need for services has been assessed, a plan needs to be drawn up by the practice nurse and the other members of the primary healthcare team to determine the most appropriate way to deliver those services. Resources must be considered: time, skills and finances. This is known as the commissioning process. The primary healthcare team are probably best placed to commission services as they work closely with the public within the area in which they live and are able to gather information on what services are required from the practice profile (*Chapter 1*). *Primary Care – The Future* (NHS Exec, 1996) went so far as to say that primary care in Britain has always been able to deliver services as effectively as possible within the resources available. The practice nurse can use her skills to help produce protocols relevant to the plan and identify what skills are needed within practice to meet them.

The national agenda — implications for practice nurses

There have been numerous documents and strategies produced by the Government over the last ten years aimed at health professionals, most of which encourage collaboration and joint working. The most radical could arguably be, *The new NHS — modern, dependable* (DoH, 1997a). A review of most of the latest white papers, such as the *NHS Plan* (DoH, 2000), *Making a difference* (DoH, 1999); and public health strategies, such as, *Smoking kills* (DoH, 1998), reveal that practice nurses hold a key role in their implementation and success. This is demonstrated in the following reviews of some of the most important white papers and strategies to be introduced in the last few years, and their impact on practice nursing.

The new NHS — modern, dependable (DoH, 1997a)

This White Paper was introduced by the Government as probably the greatest single act of modernisation ever achieved by a Labour Government (Blair, 1997) and was brought about in a bid to end GP fund-holding and the internal market. It was to introduce NHS Direct, a twenty-four-hour telephone advice line for the general public, which in turn would have implications for general practice. Some patients can now be given advice without a GP consultation, or others may be referred directly to the general practice.

Primary care groups were born from this White Paper. This chapter shows the impact that this is having on practice nursing and nursing as a whole.

Our Healthier Nation (DoH, 1997b)

Our Healthier Nation, which superseded *Health of the Nation*, holds the same principles of providing a strategy for England that will improve the health of the worst off and narrow the health divide between the classes (DoH, 1997b).

It resulted from the Acheson report and although the document suggests that health in general is improving, it also states that the divide is not.

Practice nurses have an important role to play in delivering the new agenda within this and other documents. The practice nurse's role includes ensuring that services provided are accessible to all members of society, to help make it a fairer NHS.

Practice nurses have a responsibility, along with the rest of the primary healthcare team, to tackle the targets set out in *Our Healthier Nation* (DoH, 1997b). It may be that this is done as a team, as an individual, or both (*Figure 3.1*). The main targets of *Our Healthier Nation* are:

i) To prevent accidents.
ii) Mental health — improvement of services and reduction in suicides.
iii) Reducing the incidence of coronary heart disease/stroke.
iv) Reducing the incidence of cancers.

NHS Plan (DoH, 2000)

One of the most recent papers to be released is the *NHS Plan* (DoH, 2000). This was introduced to address and tackle problems, including access to services. The plan was introduced along with the promise of extra funding for the NHS to help to implement and sustain the principles within it.

The ten core principles of the plan provide promises of how the NHS will deliver its services over the next few years, these include partnership and performance in the NHS professions and the wider NHS workforce, patient care and prevention.

The plan holds many implications and opportunities for practice nursing which are demonstrated by *Figure 3.2*, along with the expectations that patients may have regarding services provided by the practice nurse in the future.

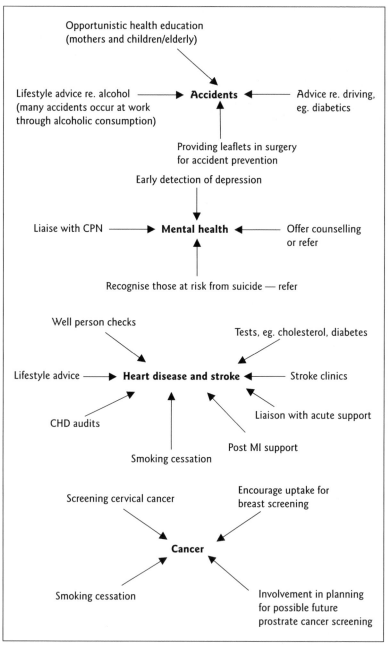

Figure 3.1: How can practice nurses contribute to achieving the targets of *Our Healthier Nation*

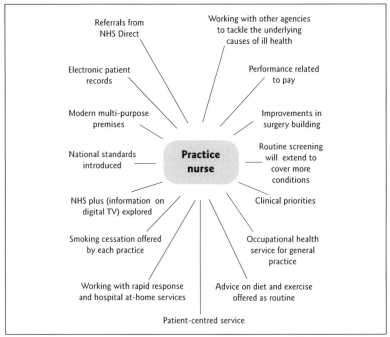

Figure 3.2: Implications of the *NHS Plan* (DoH, 2000) for practice nurses

The plan clearly has implications for the workload of practice nurses with many arguing that their workload will increase dramatically, for instance, it entails introducing new screening programmes. Some of the areas of care have already been taking place in practice and others may serve to improve the care that is given. There is also a strong emphasis in the plan that the service should be patient-centred and this has implications when planning and delivering services. The plan recommends that the practice population, ie. the service users, should be involved (*Chapter 5*).

Making a Difference (DoH, 1999)

Among the Government's ambitious programmes designed to improve the NHS, health and the inequalities in health, are plans to include the contribution of nursing, midwifery and health visiting.

Making a Difference (DoH, 1999) sets out the Government's intentions for the nursing profession, taking into account the results from consultations around the country from nurses, midwives and health visitors.

The document gives details of the numbers of nurses, midwives and health visitors in practice, demonstrating that they are the largest staff group and group of healthcare professionals in the NHS.

It recognises that the context of care and the population of the United Kingdom is changing and that nursing needs to respond to this. It acknowledges that practice nurses, specifically, are an important part of primary care and discusses the opportunities for those nurses to develop new ways of addressing the needs of the population with innovative schemes (such as primary care services' pilots).

The document illustrates eleven key sections, some of which are shown in *Table 3.3*, in relation specifically to practice nursing.

Table 3.3: *Making a Difference* (DoH, 1999) — the implications for practice nursing

1.	Making a difference + practice nurses	Improving people's health and lives High quality care through research and audit
2.	New nursing in the NHS + practice nurses	Support in community for those suffering from chronic illnesses Practice nurse as part of an integrated team providing continuity of care Using Internet to gain up-to-date information Involving the public in decision making
3.	Recruiting more nurses + practice nurses	Visits to schools for career's days
4.	Education and training + practice nurses	Theory/practice gap bridged ENB courses developed and improved Partnership between mentors and educational establishment Involved in planning and delivery of training

Smoking Kills (DoH, 1998)

This document makes up yet another piece of the jigsaw of Government strategies and policies for improving people's health and, like all the others, has implications for practice nursing.

Smoking is now reported as the principle avoidable cause of premature deaths in the UK (DoH, 1998), killing 120,000 people per year. It has been accused of affecting the health and even killing people who do not smoke — 'passive smoking' — as well as those who do.

This White Paper plays an important part in improving health by setting out proposals to help people who wish to give up smoking. Many primary care groups are investing money in resources and training for practice nurses to enable them to become involved in smoking cessation.

Figure 3.3 shows the relationship between the document and practice nursing and demonstrates the part that practice nurses can play in reducing smoking and smoking-related deaths.

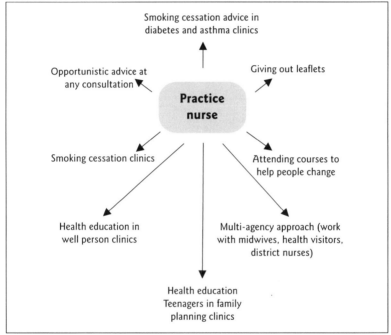

Figure 3.3: *Smoking Kills* (DoH, 1998) — The role of the practice nurse

Assessing health needs

Along with the many documents cited above, according to the recent *NHS Plan* (DoH, 2000), assessing health care effectively and correctly is a very important function of the NHS. There is little point in providing a service that is not needed or one that is not addressing the needs of the people to whom it is meant to serve.

There are three areas of healthcare need that affect the way that services are planned, these are:

1.   Clinical needs of the individual patients within the practice.

2. Healthcare need when planning services for the practice population.
3. Healthcare need when planning services for the PCG.

A practice nurse working within a small population within a primary care group must strike a balance between the needs of the individual patients and the needs of the population as a whole. It is important that individual needs are considered; it is also important that the practice nurse feeds back to the primary care group board the particular needs of that practice in order that they be considered in the local planning and commissioning of health care. It must be remembered that if patients are asked to make 'wish lists' of their needs and expectations, that these lists are likely to be lengthy, which may not be easily matched by the natural limits on resources.

Individual needs of each patient can be assessed in a number of ways, either by clinical examination, interview/consultation, or questionnaires which include the physical, mental or social needs of the patient.

For example, during a consultation an asthma patient may admit to having a cough, feeling stressed and have a dislike of using their inhaler in public. Their needs may be assessed in the following ways:

1. By clinical examination: to assess the state of their asthma.
2. By interview: to assess their perception of asthma, the reasons for not wanting to use inhalers in public, any other reasons for feeling stressed.
3. By questionnaire: to determine factors. For example: Are appointment times suitable? If they do not attend for appointments, why? Do they suffer from any regular symptoms? What type of service do they want/expect from the practice? Their opinions regarding treatment.

The resulting intervention may be as simple as providing a trained asthma nurse to advise on appropriate treatment, thus reducing the symptoms and so the patient would not need to use his inhalers as much in public.

If the need for an asthma clinic or an asthma-trained nurse is identified, it may be necessary to accommodate training for the practice nurse to deliver the service. The cost effectiveness of this has also to be considered, after all, it is a waste of resources to provide the service for just a few people.

Responding to health needs does not only include services provided by the health service, but also other agencies should be considered. For instance, it benefits the asthma patient if smoking in his workplace is prevented by introducing non-smoking zones.

In the above scenario, the following are important to meet the needs of the asthma patient:

1. A health professional available to the practice who is trained in asthma.
2. Access to the asthma clinic/health professional by the patient.
3. Choice between inhaler devices.
4. Education of the public in the acceptance of asthma in order to reduce stigma.

It can be seen that from one patient alone at least four health needs have been identified.

When planning the services in response to those needs, a general decision-making process concerned with managing change, can be used by a practice nurse. *Figure 3.4* shows a simple but effective framework to use when planning health care and services. This can form a cycle, to readdress health needs as regularly as needed (Edwards *et al*, 1994).

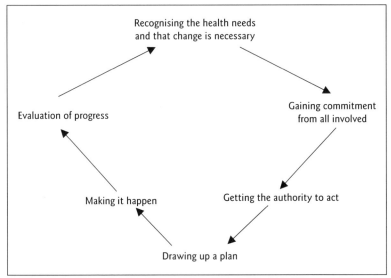

Figure 3.4: Assessing healthcare needs by adapting a model for the management of change

A Health Improvement Programme (HImP), is a five-year plan of action drawn up by the stakeholders of primary care (health authority, PCG, trusts, public, dentists, pharmacists, etc.). The aim of the plan is to identify priorities for action by these parties so that they can be addressed.

The programmes were set up by the Government in April, 1999, in a bid to replace the internal market set up by the previous government. The HImPs are implemented at local levels by the health authorities in partnership with PCGs and PCTs and revised annually to comply with new guidance. They should also operate within National Service Frameworks.

There are five strategic themes which form the basis of HImPs (*Table 3.4*).

Table 3.4: Five strategic themes of a health improvement programme

1.	Public health and inequalities in health
2.	Range and location of health and relevant social services
3.	Government's medium-term financial strategy for public services
4.	National Frameworks for assessing performance
5.	Involving patients and the public in planning and monitoring services

Baker, 2000

Due to the very nature of health improvement programmes, there are many examples which differ around the country. These include; prevention of heart disease, cancer services, children's services and mental health services.

Health action zones

As a result of an announcement in June, 1997 by the Secretary of State for Health, Frank Dobson, health action zones (HAZs) have been established in areas of deprivation to tackle the problems associated with poor health and deprivation.

Health action zones were another initiative in the Government's bid to reduce inequalities in health. The action plan for HAZs usually involves local communities, the voluntary sector, local businesses and health service bodies working together to develop projects, initiatives and services for people of their community.

The proposals of at least ten HAZs in April, 1998 were to address three strategic objectives:

- to identify and address the public health needs of local areas
- to increase the effectiveness, efficiency and responsiveness of the service
- to develop partnership for improving people's health and relevant services (Cook, 1998).

HAZ status was awarded in response to bids from health authorities around Britain, following guidance from the NHS Executive letter (EL(97)65). As part of the bid health authorities and the new primary care groups have to give short, medium and long-term objectives of their project. Dobson hoped that HAZ pilots would help to test new models of health care in order that they may be used in other areas of the country.

It is relevant for practice nurses to understand the objectives for HAZs and to know whether their practice falls within an area for development, as they hold the knowledge, skills and ability to be innovative and contribute to its success.

The action plan for HAZs usually involves local authorities and communities as well as health professionals in developing projects, initiatives and services for the people of that community.

Conclusion

This chapter has cited only a few documents and no doubt others will be following. By examining the issues it becomes apparent that practice nursing has an important part to play within the Government's national agenda and the public health domain. It is vital that practice nurses build up a strong voice by networking with each other and forming focus groups. This will enable them to influence national policy by contributing and commenting towards future documents and plans.

4

Skills required in the developing role

Introduction

As well as the clinical skills and competencies needed for the role of practice nurse, it is important to be able to communicate effectively with other professionals and the patient. This chapter examines the art of communication and how it may serve to influence the nurse/patient relationship.

If practice nursing is to remain at the forefront of primary care, it is necessary that it manages effectively all the changes happening within it (*Chapter 3*), and does not just survive them.

Communication

We can greatly increase the efficiency of our communicating with the benefit to the productiveness of our work and the enjoyment of our relationships.

Nolan, 1989

Communication is the essence of our very survival, even the most primitive of animals need to communicate in order to exist. It seems surprising that this skill, on which we rely so much, is very rarely taught as part of our education. Health professionals have reported feeling inadequately trained to communicate with patients and, despite communication being part of the British undergraduate medical education, patients still complain about poor communication and inadequate information giving (Sowden *et al*, 2001).

The way in which we communicate as human beings is important: how often have people said something that they almost straight away wish that they had not, how often have we heard of people 'getting the wrong end of the stick', or of saying something but meaning something else?

Tanner (1976) defined communication between individuals as the process of creating a meaning. Communication is a vital component of the practice nurse's role, be it verbal or non-verbal, illustrated by the many times that an appointment consists of no more than sitting and discussing a problem or an issue with no physical intervention taking place. This can be just as effective and useful to the patient as an intervention, such as an operation or procedure.

Practice nurses and other nurses use communication skills in all areas of their work, both verbal and non-verbal, suggesting that communication should be an important part of nurse education both pre- and post-registration.

Dr Fritz Schumacher (1987) described the four steps that he considered were involved when one person wishes to communicate with another. These are:

❖ The speaker must know, with some precision, what the thought is that he wishes to convey.

❖ He must find visible (including audible) symbols; gestures, bodily movements, words, intonation, etc., which in his judgement are able to 'externalise his 'internal' thought; this may be called the first translation'.

❖ The listener must have a faultless reception of these visible symbols. He must accurately hear what is being said, knowing the language used, and accurately observe the non-verbal symbols (such as gesture and intonation) that are being employed.

❖ The listener must then in some way integrate the numerous symbols he has received and turn them into thought; this may be called the 'second translation'.

Using this as an example, it can be seen that any interruption to any of the first stages will result in communication between the practice nurse and the patient failing. This illustrates that the listener (patient) is as much a part of the communication process as the speaker (practice nurse). The practice nurse must set the level of communication against the knowledge and understanding of the patient, using language that they will understand. This can be highlighted in four stages:

❖ Firstly, the practice nurse needs to understand the nature of the problem that the patient has booked in to see her about. That is not to say that the problem written down in the appointment book by the receptionist should be taken for granted. The patient may not have wished to convey the exact nature of their problem when booking, on the other hand, sometimes a written message can be misinterpreted. For instance, if 'rubella' was written it could be interpreted in a number of different ways: the patient thinks that they have rubella, is worried about catching rubella, needs a blood test for rubella status or requires a rubella vaccine. Communication and interpretation are so important.

❖ Secondly, the practice nurse needs to plan the best way visibly to get advice or thoughts over to the patient. This may include words, leaflets, aids or models (eg. model airway to demonstrate asthma), and body movements (eg. demonstrating the best way to insert eye drops).

❖ Thirdly, the patient must be able to observe non-verbal symbols and accurately hear what is being said.

❖ Lastly, to ensure that the third stage has been achieved the practice nurse should check that the listener has understood by making sure that the patient has received the information and turned it into thought. The practice nurse may ask the patient to repeat the information, advice or demonstration.

To communicate effectively enough time is needed to pass through all four stages: to prepare, to communicate, to listen, to verify. It is important that any consultation booked with the practice nurse should be given adequate time. It would serve no purpose if only the first two stages of the communicating process took place, and for the practice nurse to send the patient home without being sure that they have understood the consultation and whether it has benefited them.

Table 4.1 shows an example of the types or methods of communication that practice nurses may be expected to use.

Table 4.1: Methods of communication

Patient records	In order for information regarding the patient to be passed on to others within the practice who may see the patient
Co-op cards	Between patient/primary care/secondary care
Memorandum	Internally between professionals
E-mail	To other professionals on IT network
Books/journals	To disseminate information to other professionals
Demonstrations	To patients/carers/relatives or other professionals
Body language	In consultation/meetings/between colleagues
Teaching	Patients/public/other professionals
Spoken word	To anyone with whom the practice nurse comes into contact
Letters	To patient/hospital/colleagues

Some methods of communication such as letters, memos, etc. may be misinterpreted. The following memo sent to the receptionists of a general practice gives an example of this.

Memo

Mrs Smith will not be seen by the district nurse on Saturday.

Can you please arrange something else?

Does this mean that Mrs Smith does not wish to be seen by the district nurse, does not wish to be seen on Saturday, or does it mean that she will not be seen because the district nurses are unavailable?

Whenever possible, face-to-face communication is favourable and less likely to be misinterpreted.

As changes are introduced within primary care it is important to communicate with the rest of the primary healthcare team to enable those changes to be managed and implemented in the most effective way, and secure the delivery of high quality care to the public.

Managing change

> *There is nothing more difficult to carry out, nor more*
> *doubtful of success, nor more dangerous to handle, than to*
> *initiate a new order of things.*
>
> Machiavelli, cited by Nolan, 1990

Those practice nurses, who are at the leading edge of primary care and who embrace changes to enable the service to be improved, need to understand the principles of managing and encouraging change within the primary healthcare team. Such principles may be learnt not only from models used in health care, but also from experience outside of health care, eg. industry and commerce. As the emphasis on care shifts from secondary to primary care, practice nurses are going to have to learn to cope with and manage such changes. Those nurses who like to go to work in the morning, do the same job that has always been done, and go home in the evening will not last in today's primary care-led NHS. Nolan (1989) highlights this:

> *You do what you have always done but you don't get what*
> *you always got.*

The principles behind managing change have been used in a number of ways, especially through health promotion. Practice nurses along with other health professionals have used the model by Prochaska and Diclemete (1984) for a number of years. Often known as the transtheoretical model it follows five stages of behaviour change from the pre-contemplation stage through to maintenance where the client has managed to change their behaviour and is able to maintain it reasonably well (Birmingham Specialist Community Health Trust Health Promotion Service [BSCHT HPS], 2000).

The practice nurse is involved in primary, secondary and tertiary care, which means that they come into contact with patients who are well or who show potential risks of disease, as well as patients suffering from a particular disease. In addition, the practice nurse, usually through familiarity, has a good rapport with the patient, giving her the ideal opportunity to negotiate behavioural change on a one-to-one basis. Consultations, such as 'well person' checks and over-75 health-checks, provide an ideal opportunity to exercise skills in health promotion. The practice nurse is also in a very good position to audit and evaluate any progress in behavioural change, as she may well see the patient at every visit and be able to make comparisons from the last consultations.

Change and experimenting with change are vital to the health service for several reasons. It gives nurses a chance to identify new possibilities, some of which may be an improvement on what is already happening. In some instances, a procedure that has been carried out in the same way for years may not be getting as good a result as was first experienced. This could be due to a number of reasons: the changing environment, an increase in people's expectations, improvement in products, or audit and research may prove that there is a more effective alternative.

Changes within nursing should be viewed as an opportunity and not a threat. The new knowledge obtained from each change made can be used to minimise the risks of the next. For example, if a practice nurse wished to introduce a new method of addressing the problem of non-attenders in her practice, she may start off with those who do not attend a particular clinic, for example, a well man clinic. This would ensure that the system was effective before moving on to tackle other areas where non-attendance was a problem.

Change and experimenting within general practice also encourages innovation and new ideas, which may be disseminated to other practices as an example of good practice. Mistakes or change that have been ineffective should not be considered a failure, merely a learning tool. These instances may be disseminated, using the many methods of communication (*Table 4.2*) as a tool for other practices to learn from and prevent others from making the same mistake.

As mentioned earlier, the nurse working within general practice has a number of different disciplines of people to consider when introducing and managing change. The changes may affect ancillary staff, administration staff, practice managers, general practitioners and the rest of the primary healthcare team. When managing change, the practice nurse should create an environment that encourages change and experimenting and plan before any change is made. Ideally, the change being introduced should have the full support of the practice staff, managers, general practitioners and the primary healthcare team in order to reduce resistance. Some people have a fear of change for a number of reasons, including fear of the unknown or associated fears such as an increase in workload. Oldcorn (1996) examined the management of change and came up with a few theories on how to reduce resistance. These have been adapted in *Table 4.2*.

Table 4.2: Reducing resistance to change

❖ The change needs to have the full commitment of the practice manager and staff, general practitioners, primary healthcare team and maybe even the PCG

❖ The change is more acceptable if you involve the practice and primary healthcare team from the beginning, and come up with the management of change as a team decision if possible

❖ It helps if the change is going to reduce workloads and increase patient care within the team

❖ The change should not threaten roles or jobs within the group. An example of the threat of role erosion has been experienced within the introduction of integrated nursing teams and may possibly be a factor in the breakdown of some of them

❖ Changes that should be interesting and exciting will meet less resistance

❖ Changes brought about with the consideration of others' values and ideals will meet less resistance

❖ If influencing managers, general practitioners or PCGs, an economic incentive may reduce resistance to the changes planned

Adapted from Oldcorn, 1996

One of the major changes that have occurred within general practice over the last decade was the introduction of nurse-led clinics. As the emphasis on care has shifted from secondary to primary care, GPs have experienced an increase in workload, and they have had to examine how best the care can be managed within the practice. There has been an increase in nurse-led clinics such as asthma, diabetes, well person, etc. and, in some practices, nurses are managing minor illness clinics and triage. A practice nurse may well be expected to develop an existing clinic or service or start from scratch.

Setting up nurse-led clinics

When planning to set up a clinic there are a number of considerations to keep in mind. The first step is to identify a need for the service.

1. The practice computer or disease register will give an indication of patient age and morbidity to ensure that there are enough patients needing the service. A comparison with national data will also indicate whether there is a deficit in the number of patients diagnosed or identified with certain conditions

(eg. asthma effects approximately 15% of the population [National Asthma and Respiratory Training Centre, 1998] therefore a list size of 5,000 should identify approximately 750 patients). The practice nurse needs to plan for the estimated number of patients likely to need the service and prioritise them in order to plan who to invite first. It would be difficult for the practice nurse to be able to consult with 750 asthma patients effectively in a short time, so the patients to be invited first may be those who are on medication and have not been seen at all to review their asthma, and/or those who have needed emergency treatment in the last few months.

2. Once the need for a clinic or service has been identified, the next step is to plan how the clinic will be run and consider questions such as, 'is the service best provided from the practice premises, or could it be delivered to the patients' home or from other venues?' If the service is probably best delivered from the practice it may be the responsibility of the practice nurse to organise and develop it. After identifying the need for a clinic or service it is important to determine whether there are any local or national criteria or existing programmes in place before launching it. If there are, the principles or protocols from these may be adopted within the practice plan (*Figure 4.1*).

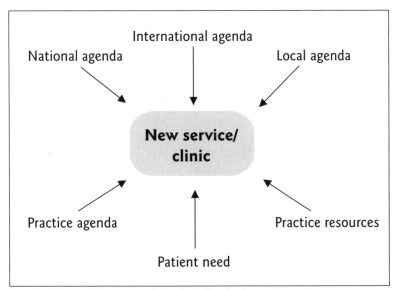

Figure 4.1: Factors to consider when developing a new service

It may be preferable to develop clinics at a set time, ie. booking in patients with the same need or illness in one block of sessions. The advantages are:

- patients and patients' relatives may meet others in a similar position and gain support
- having a set clinic enables the nurse to prepare the same equipment making it easier to use
- if all the patients booked into a clinic require advice and care for the same thing, it may be easier for the practice nurse to focus on that aspect of her role rather than having a mixed clinic or booking system
- it is easier to set aside protected time for each patient within a clinic with less opportunity for extras to be sent through for other things.

There is, however, a disadvantage of holding a clinic at a specific time. The clinic times may not suit all patients and their relatives, resulting in poor attendance.

In some practices it may be impracticable to hold set clinics (for instance, in a single-handed GP practice, or practices without adequate resources), in this case the nurse may have to be more flexible and see patients within her normal routine clinic, giving the patients more choice of times to attend. As long as enough time is allocated to their appointment this should not be a problem.

It may be appropriate in some instances to see patients without an appointment, especially if the practice has a large amount of non-attenders. It is important that appointment times are agreed between GP, reception staff and nurses to ensure that enough time is allocated to each patient to enable an appropriate consultation to take place. Of course, the very nature of general practice may involve seeing people as an emergency or opportunistically, and this may lead to the occasional delayed appointment.

When organising a clinic, or care, for a specific area it is important to ensure that all staff who are likely to be involved, including administration staff, are aware of the procedures for calling patients, booking and recalling. It is important that all staff have received adequate training for the role that they are to perform. If a practice nurse is to run a clinic without the presence of a GP, she should have received the appropriate training and be competent to do so (UKCC, 1992).

When arranging appointment times for the sessions, the content needed within the consultation should be considered. It may be considered appropriate to allocate every patient an appointment time of twenty minutes. It is inevitable that some appointment times will need to be longer than others. To expect all consultations to last five minutes is unrealistic. A patient may have booked to have their blood pressure taken, a two-minute procedure; however, research has shown that lifestyle changes can significantly reduce blood pressure and so it is as important to advise on lifestyle as well as taking the blood pressure itself. In order to take a history, discuss lifestyle and develop a patient plan, a consultation would need to be longer than five minutes. Unlike acute nursing, the practice nurse may see the same patient for a number of years and be regarded as a friend; extra time may be taken to look at the photographs of the grandchildren that may be produced inadvertently at the end of a consultation! This is a valuable part of the consultation, as it may serve to develop a rapport between nurse and patient and improve trust.

Once a clinic or service has been planned, publicity is important. If the clinic is for a chronic disease such as asthma, patient information in newsletters or posters within the waiting room may invite patients who are experiencing specific health problems, such as nocturnal cough, to visit the clinic. If the object of the clinic is for screening the 'well' population then the posters or newsletter may include an invitation to visit the practice nurse and information about the services available. The health authority or primary care group may send information leaflets to the local population, a useful media to promote the clinic.

Planning resources is vital and the clinic needs to be run in a realistic, cost effective manner. Instruments and equipment should be in working order and be regularly checked as per the manufacturer's instructions. There should be adequate room to carry out clinical procedures and the patient should have privacy at all times.

To ensure that the clinic is run to a desirable standard, research-based clinic protocols that have been agreed between GP and practice nurse should be used. Standards for the clinic or service should also be stated and audited against to ensure that the practice is providing a high quality, responsive service.

It is also good practice to plan what the audit will be measuring so that the required information is collected. The member of staff responsible for the data collection, questionnaires, etc. needs to be aware of the information needed and how it will be collected and validated. The primary care group may have members involved in auditing clinical effectiveness and they are usually willing to visit the practice with information and help if needed.

What is meant by accountability?

Accountability is like being pregnant — you cannot be slightly pregnant.

Glover, 1999

Before commencing on the first day in general practice, a practice nurse should read and apply the *Scope of Professional Practice* (UKCC, 1992) to her particular post. This protects the nurse, the employer and the general public, especially as many general practitioners are unaware of the experience and capabilities of a registered general nurse. This could indicate that some employing general practitioners might not understand the full implications of nurses carrying out tasks for which they are not competent. The practice nurse should aim to learn and become competent in a few tasks per week or month, and access any external training courses that are available to reinforce practical knowledge with theory. It may be useful to prioritise the areas of care that the practice is likely to require the nurse to be competent in. Take advantage of any formal induction course or package offered (*Chapter 1*).

Practice nursing is a dynamic and complex profession which is developing rapidly, and often results in an increase in responsibility. All nurses need to know to whom they are accountable and for whom they are responsible, and be aware of some of the basic issues in law that will guide their practice. It is essential for practising nurses to understand the importance that the UKCC and its documents holds for the safety of the professional and the public. Accountability inevitably increases as autonomy grows.

Accountability within the profession is not a new concept. In 1919, the nurse registration acts were passed as a result of the campaigning by Mrs Bedford Fenwick and the British Nursing Association. They had the aim of state registration for nurses following three years training. These acts gave rise to the General Medical Councils. Some cynics, including Florence Nightingale, were against registration, considering nursing to be a vocation not a profession. This argument is still heard from some today. However, it was not until 1979 that the Nurses, Midwives and Health Visitors Act came into force (Consulting, 1998) giving rise to the birth of the United Kingdom Central Council for Nursing, Midwifery and Health Visiting (UKCC), whose role was:

- maintaining a register of qualified nurses, midwives and health visitors
- setting standards for education, practice and conduct
- providing advice on professional standards
- dealing with cases of misconduct or unfitness to practice.

The UKCC subsequently produced many guidelines and documents, including the *Code of professional conduct* (UKCC, 1984). This was followed by a number of documents and guidelines to be used by all professional nurses, including the *Scope of Professional Practice* (UKCC, 1992). As nursing meets the new millennium the UKCC is being reformed and improved, including a change of name (the Nursing and Midwifery Council [NMC]) and its constitution.

Accountability can be defined as:

The requirement that each nurse is answerable and responsible for the outcome of his or her professional actions.

Pennels, 1997

It is recognised that as accountability and authority are interdependent, a greater degree of accountability is expected of those with greater authority. This is important when practice nurses are developing professionally into posts such as nurse practitioners and advanced nurse practitioners. The introduction of nursing consultants in the last couple of years also raises issues over accountability and responsibility.

The practice nurse is accountable in four ways to differing authorities:

- the public
- the individual patient
- the profession
- the employer.

Nurses are ultimately accountable to the patient through duty of care and common law. If nurses act negligently towards their patients then the patient may take action through the civil courts for negligence.

Accountability is also raised through contract law to their employer, which is likely to be the general practitioner but may be different in the future as practice nurses become employed by local authorities or primary care groups. If a nurse is entering general practice or any type of pilot scheme they need to establish who they are accountable to through contract law (whoever they have signed a contract with). If the nurse then acts negligently towards a patient they can also be in breach of their working contract and be sued by their employer.

The practice nurse is also accountable to the public as a whole. The public indirectly pay for healthcare services through taxation, making them a stakeholder in the service provided by the nurse. If a practice nurse acts in a way that is negligent and affects the public they can be sued under criminal law (Wilson, 1996).

The UKCC sets codes and standards for practice to protect the public and the nurse. If the negligent act is proven serious enough, the UKCC is justified in removing the practitioner's name from the register in order to protect the public.

The *Scope of Professional Practice* (UKCC, 1992) is probably one of the most important documents that the UKCC has developed. The document is meant to act as a guideline or framework for practitioners to work within. The very nature of practice nursing and role expansion means that probably no two practice nurses are working in the same way. Every practice and practice population has differing needs and priorities, so this would make it impossible for the *Scope of Professional Practice* to be prescriptive. It has, however, taken away the certificates of competence that nurses used to need. In the eighties, nurses were unable to take on any expansion to their role unless they had a certificate (usually from a doctor) to say that they were competent to do so, for example, to take blood. The *Scope of Professional Practice* allows a practitioner the freedom to expand their role safely and appropriately. The main clauses of the scope are shown in *Table 4.3*.

Table 4.3: Clauses of the *Scope of Professional Practice*

The nurse should:

1. act always in such a manner as to promote and safeguard the interests and well-being of patients and clients

2. ensure that no action or omission on their part, or within their sphere of responsibility, is detrimental to the interests, condition or safety of patients and clients

3. maintain and improve their professional knowledge and competence

4. acknowledge any limitations in their knowledge and competence and decline any duties or responsibilities unless able to perform them in a safe and skilled manner

---

UKCC, 1992

When a nurse is about to, or asked to, take on another aspect of the role that differs from their original practice it is important to find out whether that aspect of the role is appropriate and in the right context. For instance, it is not appropriate for a practice nurse to hold a clinic just to insert contraceptive implants. It is, however, appropriate to learn how to insert implants to enable the practice nurse to provide more holistic care and a comprehensive family planning service — discussing first the choice of methods and then offering a follow-up appointment. If the expansion of her role is merely a way of making more money for the practice or boosting the figures for the annual report this may be considered as an inappropriate role expansion. Of course, if it was to benefit the patients and at the same time benefit the practice this would be acceptable.

The most important aspect of role expansion and the scope of practice, especially for a nurse new to general practice, is that they are adequately trained for the post and role that they are about to undertake. Again, it is difficult to define what constitutes appropriate training, but as seen in *Chapter 1*, a comprehensive induction package is the most effective way to introduce a nurse into general practice.

An important question for any nurse to ask themselves when embarking upon a particular aspect of their role is, 'am I any good at what I am about to do?' If the answer is yes, and they have received appropriate training and education so that they are fully aware of the theoretical and practical aspects of the task, then what they say is true in a number of ways. Audit and/or patient questionnaires can provide a good indicator of the quality of care being given. Mentorship, including supervision of practice directly by another practitioner or clinical supervision, is another effective way of ensuring standards of care.

Problems can arise within practice if the nurse lacks adequate training and supervision, or if there is poor allocation of time. If a nurse has to 'fit in' patients between appointments or is allocating too short a time for routine appointments then mistakes may be made. It is good practice for the practice nurse to educate the rest of the staff and doctors regarding accountability and the importance of time allocation when giving appointments. The task of giving an immunisation may only take a few minutes but to give appropriate advice, answer questions and fill in the records correctly may take far longer.

With the introduction and development of the specialist practitioner, it is worth briefly examining accountability in relationship to those practice nurses who may be developing their role. Pennels (1998) suggested that specialists are not only accountable in the ways previously discussed, but are also accountable to the team for which they are responsible, and accountable for the delegation of tasks within that team.

Clinical supervision (*Chapter 2*) is another area of development in which the supervisor and supervisee both have accountability and responsibility. If the supervisee is seen to be a danger to the patient and the supervisor does not take any action, he /she will be held accountable. Any information disclosed within the supervision session must be followed up in an appropriate way by the supervisor or supervisee, and the principles of law regarding liability should be considered. This should be included in any ground rules or contracts drawn up before the clinical supervision sessions commence.

In summary, it is apparent that if a practice nurse is negligent towards a patient, either deliberately or ignorantly (through being unaware of the *Code of professional conduct* and the *Scope of Professional Practice*), they may lose their job. In addition, there is a possibility that they may lose their status on the professional register, be sued for negligence and end up in prison or with a fine. It is important for all induction programmes to include education on accountability and the implications of the documents provided by the UKCC for the benefit of nurses new to general practice.

Developing protocols, guidelines and standards

Protocols, guidelines and standards can contribute to the provision of a high standard of patient care, evidence-based practice and legal protection within practice nursing. It is important that they are used correctly and in the right context. Guidelines are a principle or framework that are put together to determine the course of action to be taken by a practitioner, whereas a protocol is more prescriptive. A guideline used for diabetes may state that:

> All diabetic patients should receive advice regarding foot-care at least annually.

Written as a protocol it would state:

> Each patient will have their feet examined by the practice chiropodist,

or that:

> The diabetic nurse will check for pedal pulses and signs of infection twice yearly.

A protocol is a set of instructions based on the guidelines.

Guidelines may be formulated at a national, local or practice level. Protocols should be developed at practice level for and by the practitioners involved. Standards are an 'accepted example of something by which others are judged' (Collins, 1992). In nursing this means that a level of care is agreed by those responsible for setting standards. The standard set should be considered as a minimum not a maximum standard and the aim of nursing care should be to achieve at least the set standard. The standard provides a tool for audit and re-evaluation of the care given. An example of a standard used in the care of diabetic patients could read as follows:

> Ninety per cent of all diabetic patients within the practice should have their blood glucose level monitored twice yearly.

A simple audit of the number of diabetic patients who have had blood glucose levels tested compared with the total number of patients could then be measured and compared to the standard. If the figure is below the standard of 90% then the practice needs to examine ways of improving for the following year.

Why do we need protocols?

Protocols, guidelines and standards can:

❖ Contribute towards clinical governance within practice. Clinical governance is now one of the main focuses of primary care groups. The Royal College of Nursing (1998) have described it very simply as, 'all things that help to maintain and improve high standards of patient care'.

❖ Serve to protect the employer and the employee in instances of litigation. In cases where a complaint has been filed for negligence and staff have followed their contractual obligations, standards and protocols, the employer would usually take vicarious liability for their employee (Wilson, 1996). If the practice has protocols and standards in place and has carried out regular audits this may strengthen a case against a claim for negligence (refer audit book).

❖ Provide greater autonomy in practice if developed by the practitioners who are to use them, although if they are too prescriptive they may serve to reduce individualised patient care.

Protocols may be developed by nurses, with a specialist interest in a clinical area, for use by those less knowledgeable. A nurse new to general practice may find a set of protocols, guidelines and standards useful in the initial period within practice and she may use them as a baseline to develop practice specific protocols later on.

If developed as a primary healthcare team, protocols, guidelines and standards may also serve to promote continuity of care, less duplication of work and a more holistic package of care for the patient, as well as helping to develop joint working between disciplines.

To be effective, protocols, guidelines and standards should be explicit and evidence-based (RCN, 1993). New research is being done constantly with new evidence being uncovered, which means that the documents will need updating regularly. It is a good idea to have a designated person or team within the practice to undertake this responsibility on a regular basis.

When setting out to develop protocols, guidelines or standards it may be useful to spend time planning how to go about it to prevent time wasting and duplicating existing work. If a nurse new to general practice wishes to develop guidelines or protocols, it may be advisable to seek advice from her mentor in the first instance. The following set of questions need to be answered before embarking on the development stage:

- what existing clinics (or care) are being delivered by the nurse or primary care team?
- are there any existing protocols, standards or guidelines already in use?
- who, if anyone, already has involvement in planning clinics and protocols?
- what clinics, areas of care are planned for the future?
- what members of staff are willing to be involved?

The answers to these questions will provide a foundation from which to plan the development stage. It is worth remembering that legally all staff or their representatives who are expected to follow protocols should be involved in their development and can request that they be reviewed at any time. Staff should be informed when the development stage goes ahead and given the option to be involved.

The next stage in the development of any documents that determine nursing care would be to meet with any staff involved and to examine existing documents. These may simply need amending or updating. It is pointless to reinvent the wheel; if other professionals are using documents that work well it may be worth adapting these to the individual practice's or primary healthcare team's needs.

If there are few or no guidelines or protocols in use then the practitioner will need to list the areas of existing care or clinics and prioritise them according to need. It will be impossible, unless a large group is willing to divide the workload, for one nurse to develop a number of protocols all at once. Once the protocols, guidelines or standards have been devised, the method of auditing against them will need to be decided.

What is audit anyway?

Any plan developed for service delivery needs to consider methods of measuring the outcomes of the service, to ensure that goals or objectives of the services are met. Audit can arguably be one of the most effective ways to measure outcomes. Audit can be defined as, 'the process used by health professionals to assess, evaluate and improve the care of patients in a systematic way in order to enhance their health and quality of life' (Irvine, 1991). The aims of audit as defined by Carey and Owens (1994) are to measure:

- the appropriateness of the care delivered
- the acceptability of care
- the effectiveness
- the continuity of care
- the accessibility of care
- the efficiency of care delivered.

Dorrell (1996) suggested that detailed expert audit can also give us a greater understanding of the underlying factors that influence clinical decision making and lead to variations in clinical practice.

However, health outcomes may be difficult to measure and it may be difficult to set standards. It is relatively easy to collect data on how many patients have been commenced on hormone replacement therapy (HRT), for instance, but not so easy to measure information such as the effect that the therapy has had on the quality of their life. People and practitioners also differ in their perceptions of health and the meaning of the quality of life, which results in a bias.

It is often the practice nurse's responsibility to be involved in audit, therefore it is important for a nurse new to general practice to incorporate the subject of audit into the induction period (*Chapter 1*).

Audit is a useful tool with which to provide feedback to staff involved in the care process and is used as a benchmark for other interested parties or stake holders. When the subject of audit is broached with nurses, a physical sigh can often be heard. Practice nurses' interpretation of audit is often that of an exercise that is time-consuming and labourious. In some instances, nurses do not have the resources or support to carry out audit. However, there are many advantages to carrying out audits and in the light of clinical governance they are important to ensure that the care given by the practice nurse is cost-effective, clinically effective and of a high quality.

Audit does not have to be time-consuming and most audits can be short and effective. A well-designed audit can help to identify problems and provide sound evidence for arguing for more resources, eg. training, time, equipment and money. By auditing an area where there appears to be a problem it can often identify where the problem lies and enable staff to rectify it. For example, if there seemed to be a particularly high number of complaints regarding waiting times for GPs it may be useful to audit the times that patients are waiting. This in turn may lead to the nature of consultations being audited to discover whether the patients' waiting time could be reduced by their seeing a more appropriate professional, eg. nurse, health visitor, pharmacist or whether the appointment times needed to be lengthened or shortened.

Audit can be retrospective, enabling health professionals to look back and audit what they have already done. This may be especially useful if they need results in a limited time, eg. previous smears can be audited to identify whether there has been a problem in the past. More often, audit is prospective or current which may take more time but be more appropriate, especially when a new service is being developed. It can also be used in a number of contexts, organisational or clinical, and can be done by anyone who has access to the information required. It is important that everyone who is involved with the audit is involved with the planning, kept well-informed of its progress and is involved in any changes that are made as a result. The whole process is known as the 'audit cycle' and is used for any clinical audits carried out in general practice. *Figure 4.2* gives an example of the audit cycle used for auditing the adequacy of cervical smears.

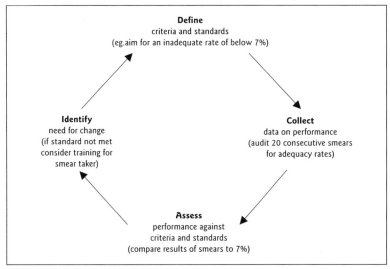

Figure 4.2: The audit cycle

Another type of audit which is a fairly new concept is 'significant events audit'. Significant events auditing is the analysing of events by the primary healthcare team, that might be considered significant in everyday practice. These events, as in critical incidents, can include both happy and critical events and have been reported to be much more flexible and enjoyable than the conventional audit. Page (2000) suggested four main courses of action possible from examining a significant event as a team, discussing the issues to ending up with an action plan:

a)   Immediate change.
b)   Further conventional audit or information gathering.
c)   No action. If a problem was dealt with correctly.
d)   Praise. People respond to positive feedback.

The process should not be used as a 'blame' tool and ground-rules regarding issues such as confidentiality and information discussed should be established first. The process of significant events auditing may also be useful as part of a clinical supervision session (*Chapter 3*).

Clinical governance

The term clinical governance is fairly new but some of the activities that go towards achieving clinical governance are not new to nursing. Clinical governance can be described as the activities, which together maintain and improve high standards of care for the patient. It has been defined by the DoH as:

> *A framework through which NHS organisations are accountable for continuously improving the quality of other services.*

Gulland, 1999

It has been introduced to tackle the variations in quality of care to prevent different services and standards being provided throughout the country and to prevent the 'postcode lottery'.

Some of the activities which are recommended for clinical governance to be implemented within practice can be seen in *Table 4.4*. It is apparent from this list that many if not all of the activities involve the practice nurse and primary healthcare team. Indeed, it is the responsibility of some practice nurses to take responsibility for clinical governance within the primary care group.

Table 4.4: Activities associated with clinical governance in practice

- ❖ Maintaining and improving clinical effectiveness
- ❖ Evidence-based medicine
- ❖ Clinical audit
- ❖ Complaints management
- ❖ Clinical leadership development
- ❖ Continuing medical education
- ❖ Continuing professional development
- ❖ Effective leadership
- ❖ Robust information
- ❖ Critical appraisal
- ❖ Safeguarding patient confidentiality

Clinical governance has been supported through a number of initiatives from the Government, including establishing the commission for health improvement (CHImp) which is responsible for reviewing NHS performance. Primary care groups and the developing primary care trusts are responsible for the implementation of clinical governance throughout Britain, and it is important for practice nurses to identify the lead person within the PCG to gain knowledge and information of strategies in their area.

There has been confusion between the terms clinical governance and clinical effectiveness. Clinical effectiveness is about doing the right things in the right way, at the right time and for the right patient (NHS Exec, 1999) — this is part of the clinical governance framework for quality.

A quality approach to healthcare is becoming more important to both providers and purchasers of health care and to the stakeholders, the patients. The quality of a product or commodity can be a difficult entity to measure. There are several definitions which all reflect the same concept, that quality is about 'the totality of features and characteristics of a product or service that bear on its ability to satisfy a given need' (Brown, 1979).

In general practice, the product or commodity on offer is the service offered by the practice from when the patient walks through the door to when they leave the practice and beyond, if they require follow-up care such as home visits or telephone advice. This means that all members of the primary healthcare team, practice staff team and the general practitioners are responsible for contributing towards this quality service. Wille (1992) supports this by saying that:

> *Quality is all about people and attitudes and not just about techniques and procedures.*

In general practice, nurses often work in isolation from other healthcare professionals and practice nurses which makes it vital to network, communicate and liaise with others.

Conclusion

It is important for the practice nurse to combine those skills and concepts discussed within this chapter with clinical competencies (*Chapter 1*) in order to develop the role and be a competent practitioner. Some of those skills may be gained from experience, learnt from peers, mentors, supervisors or by structured formal training courses.

To ensure that the practice nurse remains dynamic and delivers high quality care, the care given must be evaluated by audit, at least annually, and changed or developed accordingly.

5

The future of primary care

Introduction

This chapter examines the patient's involvement and responsibilities within the context of general practice.

To ensure that practice nursing is reacting to the needs of the public, it is necessary to be an innovative and dynamic practitioner and to develop and market the services available to ensure that they are responsive, comprehensive and competitive.

There is no doubt that the future of primary care lies not only with healthcare professionals but also with its stakeholders. The relationship with the public is becoming more important; the public are no longer considered as merely receivers of care but as stakeholders in healthcare provision and services.

Access to primary care services

Many of the Government's strategies and documents stress that access to health care, by all sectors of the community, should be improved and problems addressed. This was the purpose of the National Health Service (NHS) walk-in centres .

Nurse-led walk-in centres are being piloted and are used as 'drop-in centres', providing treatment for minor illnesses, health information and self-advice. The nature of the centres mean that they are open for longer than most GP surgeries and they accept patients from any practice, without referral. This raises concerns among some professionals that continuity of care will be lacking. It also raises questions over whether the practice, GP or practice nurse will receive feedback from the centre regarding advice given to patients. One way to overcome this would be the development of joint training programmes between members of the primary care team and the walk-in centres.

A small study by Jones (2000) discovered that in Canada women were more likely to attend walk-in clinics than men, and that children and younger adults were more likely to attend than people aged over thirty-five. If these walk-in centres were not meeting the needs of the older population this could be a valuable lesson from which to learn when planning our own services.

In many surgeries, patient participation groups contribute to the commissioning decisions when addressing the health needs of the practice. Practice nurses need to be increasingly aware of the potential role and asset of the public in this way. If patients form a strong group and can debate issues around their care, the practice is more likely to be responsive to their needs. In turn, the health authority and Government should consider their needs when planning the services that the practice should be providing.

Public involvement in primary care

No matter how well trained a practice nurse may be, or how many protocols, research and examples of good practice are followed, there is always a factor in the whole equation that is unpredictable and never conforms to text book rule — the patient! However much research or information studied by the nurse, it can never provide enough preparation for the unique questions or problems that the patients may produce.

The power of the patient should never be underestimated and despite 99% of the population responding to one kind of research-based care, it is always possible that you are going to meet Mrs 1% who does not. This again makes the role of practice nursing unique and the role of a book such as this a mere guide.

Part of the Government's plan for the future includes involving the public in health and health needs. The World Health Organization (WHO) set out the principles of primary care at the international conference of Alma Ata in 1978. Their philosophy of primary care highlighted the importance of involving the community in development, implementation and evaluation of these services. Despite this, ten years later, Ashton and Seymour (1988) argued that there was little evidence to suggest that this was happening. The present Government, another ten years later, have developed many policy directives which are meant to involve the public, but it is questionable as to what extent.

Poulton (1999) produced a paper to address whether the rhetoric of user involvement was being realised by primary healthcare services in the United Kingdom. This showed that in relation to assessing healthcare need, the vast majority of people are knowledgeable of local health needs and have realistic views of how these may be addressed. This seems to suggest that practice nurses, along with the rest of the primary healthcare team, need to listen to patients and the public when planning services. The public need to be prepared for this role and Williamson (2000) recommended that their training must be addressed along with the health professionals' so that they all know how and what they are expected to contribute.

The Government has recognised that the role of the public is a significant one. The NHS is paid by the taxes of the people and, at the end of the day, we would all expect first class health care should we need it. When developing primary care groups the Government's directives stated that:

> *Each primary care group will be required to: ... have clear arrangements for public involvement including open meetings...*

NHS, 1998

The document also cites six reasons as to why the NHS should include user and public involvement (*Table 5.1*).

Table 5.1: Why user and public involvement?

1. To contribute to greater openness and accountability in the NHS

2. To develop a greater local understanding of the issues involved in major local service changes

3. To help strengthen public confidence in the way major changes in local health services are planned

4. To develop a greater sense of local ownership and commitment to health services

5. To lead to better quality and more responsive services through listening to and understanding the needs and wishes of the health service users and involving them in service planning, development and monitoring

6. To enable local people to have access to better information about health and health services which can lead to more appropriate use of health services

Since the birth of the nursing process a few years ago, patients were more and more involved in the planning and outcomes of their own care in the secondary care setting. Now the patients and public are not only being involved in their own care in the primary and secondary care sector, but also in planning healthcare services for the whole population. As a result of the above directives, the public already have representation on primary care group boards and other members of the public are invited to all public meetings. It is the responsibility of the practice nurses to encourage the patients and their families to attend such events and become involved in their care, so that they gain autonomy, empowerment and/or a voice.

Patient empowerment

Empowerment is the sense of freedom to do something significant in changing one's life (Johns and Freshwater, 1998). This seems to suggest that for patients to become empowered they need to have significant involvement in their own health care.

Patients figure high in the Government's agenda for health. The *NHS Plan* (DoH, 2000) states that people should be at the centre of their care plan and nurses and other healthcare providers should be seen not just as care givers but as information brokers. It could be argued that for nurses to empower patients they themselves need to be empowered. Chavasse (1992) agreed with this when stating that empowerment is a state arising from valuing others and no one can value others unless they value themselves.

In general practice, the practice nurse is in the best position to make sure that the patients are empowered as they often have a unique professional relationship with the patients and their families. Practice nurses also need to decide whether it is appropriate and manageable to tailor the nursing care to each individual patient or plan care for the majority. It is the role of the practice nurse and other members of the primary healthcare team to encourage patients to take an active role in the care that they receive, and not just accept what the professionals tell them they should be doing. Along with empowerment should come some element of responsibility from the patient or client and their relatives or carers.

It is important to consider protocols, guidelines and standards of practice and work within these when planning an individual plan (*Chapter 4*), but it is also worth considering this when developing protocols and to make them flexible and not too prescriptive to allow for individuality. It may be difficult in a busy surgery environment for a practice nurse to give enough time to tailor the care to each individual, but packages of care can be produced that allow flexibility if needed. For instance, if a package of care involved reviewing the patient every six months and the patient felt more comfortable with being reviewed every four months, this may be written in to a personal care plan without causing too much extra work.

Practice nurse utilises	+	Patient has		Result	
Advice	D	Needs		P	E
Skill	I	Expectations		L	M
Knowledge	S	Aspirations	A	C	P
Time	C	Understanding	N	A	O
Support	U	Beliefs		R	W
Education	S	Culture	O	E	E
Experience	S	Social status	F		R
Financial resources	I	Health status			M
Equipment	O	Education			E
Literature/leaflets	N	Ability/disability			N
					T

Figure 5.1: Model of patient empowerment in general practice

It must be remembered that not every patient may wish to be empowered, some patients take on the 'illness' role and would rather be told by a professional, who they trust, what to do. The above model shows how the process is two-way: both patient and nurse need to consider each other's background, experience and abilities. The difficulties of empowerment may arise within this process when a patient requests care or drugs that are not endorsed by the National Institute for Clinical Excellence (NICE) or are not provided locally or approved by the primary care group. The practice nurse, practice and patient have to be realistic about the needs that may be met once the care plan has been decided. The practice nurse must also consider when planning a package of care the logistics of the package when put into practice, eg. are there enough appointment times at the appropriate time, is the patient able to contact someone if that is what the plan states?

Innovations and future practice

As the role and boundaries of practice nursing extend and the government directives and pilots become less prescriptive, the opportunities to introduce innovative practice increase.

The introduction of personal medical services (PMS) pilots in 1997 have enabled nurses to explore alternative ways of providing services in the community. The Government recommended that for a pilot to be effective it should follow the principles of good primary care. The main objectives for the pilots are:

- to promote high quality services for patients across the country
- to provide opportunities and incentives for primary care professionals to use their skills to the full
- to provide more flexible employment opportunities to primary care.

The Government invites professionals and/or practices to submit a proposal for PMS pilot status through their health authority. The proposals should meet all the criteria above while still providing services that patients are entitled to receive under general medical services (GMS).

There are over 250 PMS pilot schemes set up around the country with more planned in a third wave this year. When studying the pilot schemes, Walsh *et al* (2000) found that there were various models throughout the country, almost two hundred of them involving general practice and the rest within new structures. All of the pilots have involved innovative practice by the professionals involved, many of these being practice nurses. It is useful to explore how an innovative idea may be taken and developed. One innovative project targeted homeless people (Harrison, 1998) and provided a drop-in centre for a group who traditionally had not received a service. Others include nurse-led deep vein thrombosis and cellulite clinics and drug abuse advice (Lipley, 1999).

The Government encourages innovative practice and offers cash incentives to practices and other areas of health care which achieve improved care for their patients. The NHS learning network was developed to support the agenda of the NHS and to spread good practice in service delivery and management. The Beacon Network serves to achieve this by awarding 'Beacon status' to practices willing to take an active part in helping others nationally to improve their services. It is pointless trying to re-invent the wheel. The publication, *NHS Beacon Learning Handbook* and the web sites are updated regularly and serve as a reference, holding information about innovative practice and the ways of accessing information and observing that practice. Practice nurses who identify particular problems within their practice or primary healthcare group, may benefit from visiting or contacting a beacon site where steps have already been taken steps to address the problem.

The following framework for innovation (*Figure 5.2*), demonstrates how new practice can be achieved and the contributing factors to consider when introducing a new idea.

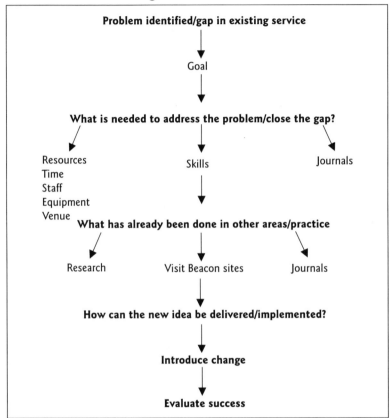

Figure 5.2: Framework for innovation

Marketing the service and oneself

As practice nurses are able to practise more autonomously and as the political gates open further to encourage new and innovative ways of working, the opportunities for professional development increase. Practice nursing is a very valuable commodity which should be marketed to reach its full potential. Marketing is not a new concept in industry and manufacturing: there is a product to be sold and the way to sell it effectively is complex and involves planning. Healthcare marketing is a new concept and differs slightly in that there is no product to sell. The product that nurses need to market is their skill and improvement to patient care and services. The NHS can learn much from the experience and skills of manufacturing and industry and adapt these principles when marketing health care. The difference between healthcare services and manufacturing is that, unlike in private industry, there is no profit to be made; however, the profit may be defined as the improved health of the population.

There are many definitions of what marketing is, Drucker (1979) states that, 'true marketing starts from the customers, their demographics, related needs and values'. Although Drucker was relating this to selling products for a profit, it bears many similarities to health care and the nurse's approach to healthcare assessment, with the customers being our public.

Ries and Trout (1989), again referring to manufacturing, suggest that marketing, 'tries to match the firm's resources and capabilities to customers' changing needs and wants at a profit'. In relation to health care, 'profit' may be considered as patient satisfaction and/or an improvement in health.

As has been discussed in previous chapters, practice nurses have many skills and much experience, all of which is marketable. The personal development plan (*Chapter 2*) lends itself to practice nursing to allow the nurse to identify the skills and experience which may in future be marketed.

Marketing may be done by the practice nurse independently promoting her own skills and expertise, or on behalf of her employer.

To enable a practice nurse to market skills it is important to know what marketing involves. It is not merely the selling of a product or skill. Marketing involves market research, identifying targets and target audiences, identifying the product and price and publicising.

It is important to know what factors affect marketing as these make a difference to the strategy. Factors include:

❖ The environment: If the area where the nurse intends to market a service is rural this will affect the client group and the marketing. For instance, people may have problems of access if a central service is to be provided, offering an opportunity for community-directed services to be developed, again, 'meeting needs of the client'. On the other hand, if the nurse works in an inner city environment the needs of the public are going to be totally different.

❖ Transport: This may not be such a problem, however health needs may be different due to the high incidence of pollution and the related diseases. Economics may also affect the service that is provided. If there is a high incidence of unemployed people the related health problems, eg. high suicide rates, CHD, etc. may need a different approach to the health needs of a higher class population (Townsend and Davidson, 1992).

❖ Social changes: These also affect marketing and the service that one would consider providing. For instance, if the healthcare service was to be provided within an area where reduction in teenage pregnancies was a priority.

❖ Political and legal changes: The last political changes brought about many opportunities for nurses to develop nurse-led services; changes in politics could just as easily affect these services, although hopefully not.

The future is bright

Over the last decade practice nurses have been able to extend their role both clinically and managerially and are carving a very exiting future for practice nursing.

There have been opportunities to become partners in health teams and some have become partners in general practice with general practitioners. The introduction of primary care groups has set a precedent for practice nurses to become involved in the assessment and planning of healthcare needs, and the Primary Care Act pilots have given them the opportunity to address those needs in a new and innovative way. Information technology in nursing has also opened up many opportunities for progress and a more efficient service.

Practice nurses are faced with enormous challenges to grasp these opportunities and make sure that health care is shaped in future to address the real needs of the population, while providing a satisfying and cost effective service. It is encouraging to see many nurses entering general practice and they, along with existing practice nurses, should join those professionals who are already making practice nursing the fulcrum of primary care.

References

Ashton J, Seymour H (1988) *The New Public Health*. Open University Press, Buckingham

Ashton J, Seymour H (1990) *The New Public Health*. Open University Press, Milton Keynes

Atkin K, Lunt N (1993) *Nurses Count: A National census of practice nurses*. Social Policy Research Unit, University of York

Atkin K, Lunt N (1995) *Nurses in Practice: The role of the practice nurse in primary health care*. Summary Report SPRU, University of York

Atkins S, Murphy K (1994) Reflective Practice. *Nurs Standard* **8**(39): 49–56

Baker M (2000) What's it all about? *Nurs Standard* **14**(16): 25

Birmingham Specialist Community Health Trust Health Promotion Service (2000) *Smoking Information in Primary care: Information pack for health care professionals*. BSCHT HPS, Birmingham

Blair T (1997) *The new NHS — modern, dependable* Executive Summary. Department of Health Publication. HMSO: 3

Bolden K, Tackle B (1984) *Practice Nurse Handbook*. 2nd edn. Blackwell Scientific Publications, Oxford: 151

Boyd EM, Fales AW (1983) Reflecting learning: key to learning from experience. *J Humanistic Psychol* **23**(2): 99–117

Bradley A (1998) *Research: Introducing a nurse into general practice*. Unpublished dissertation for BSc Hons, Primary Care, Wolverhampton University: 48

Bradshaw J (1998) Defining 'competency' in nursing (Part ll): an analytical view. *J Clin Nurs* **7**(2): 103–11

Brown T (1979) *Understanding BS5750 and other quality systems*. Gower Publishing, Aldershot

Burdett H (1893) *Hospitals and Asylums of the World*. Vol III. J & A Churchill, London

Butterworth T, Faugier J (1992) *Clinical Supervision: a position paper*. School of Nursing Studies, University of Manchester

Carey L, Owens L (1994) *Getting Started in Audit*. Magister distance learning system. RCN Publishing, London: 5

Cavanagh SJ (1993) *Orem's Model in Action*. Macmillan Publishers Ltd, London: 3

Chavasse JM (1992) New dimensions of empowerment in nursing and challenges. *J Adv Nurs* **17**(1): 1–2

Collins (1992a) *Concise Dictionary and Thesaurus*. Harper Collins, Glasgow: 469

Collins (1992b) *Concise Dictionary and Thesaurus*. Harper Collins. Glasgow: 712

Cook R (1998) Action stations. *Nurs Standard* **12**(23): 18

Cronenwett L (1983) Helping and nursing models. *Nurs Res* **32**(6): 342–6

Department of Health (1986) *The Health of the Nation*. HMSO, London

Department of Health (1990) *Working for Patients*. HMSO, London

Department of Health (1993) *A Vision for the Future*. HMSO, London

Department of Health (1997a) *The new NHS — modern, dependable*. DoH, London

Department of Health (1997b) *Our Healthier Nation, Reducing Health Inequalities: An action report.* DoH, London

Department of Health (1997c) *Shared Contributions, Shared Benefits: The report of the working group on public health and primary care.* DoH, London

Department of Health (1998) *Smoking Kills: A white paper on tobacco.* The Stationery Office, London

Department of Health (1999) *Making a Difference: Strengthening the nursing, midwifery and health visiting contribution to health and health care.* DoH, London

Department of Health (2000) *NHS Plan: A plan for investment, a plan to reform.* The Stationery Office, London

Department of Health (2000) *A health service of all the talents: developing the NHS workforce.* DoH, 2000

Diers D, Molde S (1982) Nurses in primary care: The new gatekeepers. *Am J Nurs* **83**: 742–5

Dorrell Rt Hon S (1996) *Promoting Clinical Effectiveness: A Framework for action in and through the NHS.* NHS Executive, 10 January: 31

Drucker P (1979) *Management.* Pan Books, London: 3

Edwards P, Jones S (1994) *Business and Health Planning for General Practice.* Radcliffe Medical Press, Oxford: 23

Ellis N, Chisholm J (1993) *Making Sense of the Red Book.* 2nd edn. Radcliffe Medical Press, Oxford: x

Finch J (2000) Interprofessional education and teamworking: A view from the education providers. *Br Med J* **321**(4): 1138–40

Fry J (1992) *General Practice — The facts.* Radcliffe Medical Press, Oxford: 3, 51

Gallen D (2000) *Practice Professional Development Plans.Update. A practical aid to get you started on your PDP.* Reed Business Information, Oxford: 2

Galvin K (1999) Investigating and implementing change within the primary health care nursing team. *J Adv Nurs* **30**(1): 238–47

Gibbs G (1988) *Learning by Doing: A guide to teaching and learning methods.* Further Education Unit, Oxford Brookes University, Oxford

Glover D (1999) Accountability. *Nursing Times Monographs.* Number 27. Emap Healthcare Ltd, London: 11

Gulland A (1999) What is clinical governance? *Nurs Times* **95**(9): 17

Harrison S (1998) Nurses take lead in homeless project. *Nurs Standard* **12**(21): 7

Hart E (1996) Action research as a professionalizing strategy: issues and dilemmas. *J Adv Nurs* **23**: 454–61

Hutchby P (1996) *Report on the Public Health of Wolverhampton.* Wolverhampton Health Authority, Wolverhampton

Irvine D, Irvine S (1991) *Making Sense of Audit: The business side of general practice.* Radcliffe Medical Press, Oxford: 2

Johns C (1994) Nuances of reflection. *J Clin Nurs* **3**: 71–5

Johns C, Freshwater D (1998) *Transforming Nursing through Reflective Practice.* Blackwell Science, Oxford: 52

Jones M (2000) Walk-in primary medical care centres: lessons from Canada. *Br Med J* **321**: 929

Kershaw B, Salvage J (1986) *Models for Nursing.* John Wiley & Sons Ltd, Chichester: 2

Last JM (1988) *A Dictionary of Epidemiology.* 2nd edn. Oxford University Press, Oxford

Lipley N (1999) Nursing must make most of ministers support. *Nurs Standard* **14**(9): 5

Morton-Cooper A, Palmer A (1999) *Mentoring, Preceptorship and Clinical Supervision: A guide to professional support roles in clinical practice.* 2nd edn. Blackwell Science, Oxford: 36

National Health Service Executive (1996) *Primary Care: The Future*. DoH, London

National Health Service Executive (1997) *Personal Medical Services Pilots under the NHS (Primary Care) Act 1997: A comprehensive guide*. Section 1. DoH, London

National Health Service Executive (1999) *Primary Care Trusts: Establishing better services*. NHS Exec, London: 1

National Health Service Executive (2000/2001) *NHS Beacons Learning Book*. NHS Beacon Services. Vol 1. DoH, London

Nolan V (1989) *The Innovator's Handbook: The skills of innovative management*. Sphere Books Ltd, London: 103

O'Brien M (1996) *The Case For Change: The report of the 2nd National Conference of Multi-Disciplinary Public Health, Birmingham*. 18/4 Birmingham: 3

Oldcorn R (1996) *Management*. 3rd edn. Macmillan Business Masters, Henley

Page (2000) Auditing significant events in primary care. *Community Mental Health* 2(4): 20

Pavalko, RM (1971) *Sociology of Occupations and Professions*. FE Peacock, Itasca, Illinois

Pearson A, Vaughan B (1986) *Nursing Models for Practice*. Butterworth-Heinemann Ltd, Oxford: 111

Pennels C (1997) Nursing and the law: clinical responsibility. *Prof Nurse* 13(3):162–4

Pennels C (1998) *Nursing and the Law*. Professional Nurse/Emap Healthcare, London

Plant R (1987) M*anaging Change and Making it Stick: Change starts with you*. Fontana Publishers, London: 47

Poulton B (1999) User involvement in identifying health needs and shaping and evaluating services: Is it being realised? *J Adv Nurs* 30(6): 1289–96

Prochaska J, Diclemente C (1986) Towards a comprehensive model of change. In: Miller W, Heather N, eds. *Treating Addictive Behaviours. Processes of Change*. Plenum, New York

Radford M (2000) New primary care trust invests in practice nurses. *Practice Nurse* 20(2): 66

Royal College of Nursing (1993) *Protocols and Nursing Guidance for Good Practice*. RCN Publications, London

Royal College of Nursing (1998) Improving patient care. *RCN Central Magazine*, Autumn 1998: 9

Royal College of Nursing (1999) *RCN Practice Nurse Association Handbook*. RCN Publishing Company: 6–8

Reedy B (1972) Organisation and Management: The general practice nurse. *Update* 5: 75–8

Reedy B, Metcalf AV, de Rounaine M, Newell DJ (1980) The social occupational characteristics of attached and employed nurses in general practice. *J R Coll Gen Prac* 30: 477–82

Reeves S (2000) A joint learning venture between new nurses and junior doctors. *Nurs Times* 96(38): 39

Richardson G, Maynard A (1995) *Fewer Doctors? More Nurses? A review of the knowledge base of doctor-nurse substitution*. Centre for Health Economics, University of York

Richard G, Maynard A, cited by Kernick DP (1999) Knowledge base of doctor/nurse substitution. [Discussion paper 135] York: University of York, 1995. Cited in *Br Med J* 49: 647–9

Ries E, Trout J (1989) *Bottom-up Marketing*. McGraw Hill, New York: 7

Schumacher F, cited in Nolan B (1987) *The Innovators Handbook*. Sphere Books Ltd, London: 104

Seabrook M (1998) Overcoming tribalism. *Nurs Standard* 12(20): 23

Sowden A, Forbes C (2001) On the Evidence. Patient Information. *Health Serv J* 111(5744): 36–7

Tanner B (1976) *Language and Communication in General Practice*. Unibooks, Hodder and Stoughton: 162

Townsend P, Davidson N (1992) *Inequalities in Health: The Black Report*. Penguin Books, London: 31–209

United Kingdom Central Council for Nursing, Midwifery and Health Visiting (1992) *The Scope of Professional Practice*. UKCC, London

United Kingdom Central Council for Nursing, Midwifery and Health Visiting (1992) *Code of professional conduct*. UKCC, London

United Kingdom Central Council for Nursing, Midwifery and Health Visiting (1994) *The Future of Professional Practice — The council's standards for education and practice following registration*. UKCC, London

United Kingdom Central Council for Nursing, Midwifery and Health Visiting (1995) *Position Statement on Clinical Supervision for Nursing and Health Visiting*. UKCC, London

United Kingdom Central Council for Nursing, Midwifery and Health Visiting (2001) *The PREP Handbook*. UKCC, London

Wade B (1993) The job satisfaction of health visitors, district nurses and practice nurses working in areas served by four trusts: year 1. *J Adv Nurs* **18**: 992–1004

Walsh N, Huntington J (2000) Testing the pilots. *Nurs Times* **96**(33): 32

Wille E (1992) *Quality: Achieving Excellence. Sunday Times Business Skills*. Century Press, London

Williamson C (2000) Coming on strong. *Health Service J* **16**: 26

Wilson R (1996) Who are you accountable to? *Practice Nurs* **7**(12): 29–32

World Health Organization (WHO) (1978) The Alma-Ata Conference on Primary Health Care. *WHO Chronicle* **32**

Wright SG (1986) *Building and Using a Model of Nursing*. Edward Arnold Publishers Ltd, London

Index